Upstart

Praise for *Upstart*

This admirable, clear, and powerful book brings together the voices of child development experts across the world to put a vital question on the political agenda. In Britain and former British dominions, is our outdated, inappropriate way of educating the very young harming their learning, and their lives?

Every parent, politician and bureaucrat in those countries that push children to desk-learning at younger and younger ages needs to know how much damage this will cause. And needs to embrace the less costly – in every way – approach of play-based kindergarten provision and a later school start, which works so well elsewhere.

Palmer writes in a highly readable style that conveys with ease the latest research into how children develop and grow, and what that means for their learning.

A must for anyone with children, with the care of children or with power over children's education.

Steve Biddulph, author of Raising Boys *and* Raising Girls *and many other books on parenting; psychologist; activist*

Politicians are, by and large, addicted to gross oversimplification and righteous certitude. This badly affects all of us – and most damagingly our children, who are forced, for doctrinaire and wholly unsound reasons, to start formal schooling way too early. Sue Palmer, bless her, leads the counter-charge. *Upstart* isn't liberal tosh: it is a vital reassertion of sound thinking. Buy it, read it, and give it to your MP.

Professor Guy Claxton, Emeritus Professor of Learning Sciences, University of Winchester; author of What's the Point of School?, Building Learning Power *and many other books about learning*

What could be a more important and urgent issue in the digital age than the impact of school, now and in the future, on the shaping of the twenty-first-century child's mind? Building on her wealth of experience and research, Sue Palmer presents a compelling case for reinstating the developmental needs of young children where they belong, as the most essential driving force in education policy.

Baroness Susan Greenfield, neuroscientist; broadcaster; author of The Human Brain: A Guided Tour *and many other books on the brain and consciousness*

More than ever we need to re-examine the education of children in this country – particularly in the early years – and reassert the vital place of play in children's learning. Sue Palmer, a passionate ambassador for the under-sevens, does this most convincingly. Her highly readable, challenging, carefully researched and level-headed book should be essential reading for parents and all those involved in the education of the young.

Gervase Phinn; broadcaster; education advisor; former schools inspector and professor of education; author of the Dales series of memoirs

The early years of education are all-important, as everybody knows. They are when character traits, emotional stability and intellectual curiosity should all be embedded – but too often are not. This important book is a clarion call to reconsider how we approach the education of children in these crucial years. Its challenging and radical ideas merit close study.

Sir Anthony Seldon, Vice-Chancellor, University of Buckingham; former head of Wellington College; historian; author of biographies of John Major, Tony Blair and Gordon Brown

Upstart's central message – that children flourish when they have ample opportunities to play – is at once timeless and potentially revolutionary. A critical and timely call to all adults to resist creeping 'schoolification' and protect time and space for real play in the early childhood years.

Theresa Casey, President, International Play Association

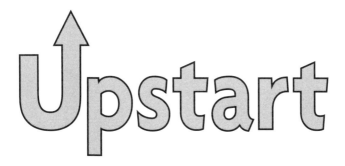

Upstart

The case for raising the school starting
age and providing what the
under-sevens *really* need

SUE PALMER

Floris
Books

First published in 2016 by Floris Books
© 2016 Sue Palmer
Sue Palmer has asserted her right under
the Copyright, Designs and Patents Act 1988
to be identified as the author of this Work
Second printing 2018

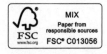

ISBN 978-178250-268-5
Printed in Great Britain
by TJ International

Contents

Summary

Why is the attainment gap in UK schools steadily widening? Why, despite endless investment in education, do we fail to shine in international surveys of literacy and numeracy? Why are doctors struggling to cope with a rising tide of mental health problems among children and young people?

A growing body of research suggests these problems all have their roots in our national attitude to early learning. For historical reasons, we expect children to start school at four or five – sitting down in a classroom to be taught reading, writing and maths – and the pressure for early academic achievement now even extends down into preschool education. It's putting many children off school from the very beginning, especially boys and those from disadvantaged backgrounds. Yet there's not a scrap of evidence that an early start on formal learning improves long-term results.

In fact, the western nations that *do* shine in international surveys have a school starting age of seven. These countries send their young children to kindergarten rather than school. Here, they're helped to acquire literacy and numeracy skills at their own rate, but the emphasis is on all-round development, health and well-being. And to support their physical, emotional, social and cognitive development, children are given plenty of opportunities to learn through their own self-directed play.

It's now well-established that active, creative, outdoor play – particularly in the early years – is vital for long-term physical and mental health. It's how nature designed young human beings to develop the self-confidence, self-control, problem-solving skills and emotional resilience they'll need to flourish in the classroom, and later, throughout their working lives.

The time has come for UK politicians to recognise the significance of play-based learning in children's earliest, most formative years. We can no longer rely on them reaping the benefits of play during out-of-school hours – over recent decades, active outdoor playtime has been replaced by sedentary indoor screen-time. And over the same period, there's been an alarming increase in developmental disorders and mental health problems.

Indeed, all the indications are that unless we change the ethos of education for the under-sevens, our children will become increasingly fragile. Rather than rushing them into ever-earlier formal learning, we must listen to experts in early child development and education, and introduce a kindergarten stage for the under-sevens.

Chapter 1
HOW DID WE GET HERE?

Why school starts so early in English-speaking nations, how politicians are now 'schoolifying' the pre-school years and why this is damaging for children and society

He's not yet five. Yesterday he was messing about in the back garden, building a 'dinosaur trap' from sticks and mud. Today he's scrubbed and shining, looking very cute in his smart new uniform but unnaturally subdued in this strange new school environment. The teacher is welcoming him into the classroom along with twenty-odd other little boys and girls: four- and five-year-old children – wide-eyed, wondering, trusting, hopeful... and so, so young!

Starting school is a big moment in anyone's life. Indeed, in today's highly competitive educational environment, it's one of the biggest moments of all – early success or failure at school is likely to affect every aspect of a child's future existence. So it would be reassuring for parents to know that the rationale underpinning the school starting policy is governed by careful consideration of young children's needs, backed up by well-established educational research, and endorsed by experts in child development.

Unfortunately, it isn't.

A very British story

In fact, starting ages for formal schooling around the world were chosen by politicians, as opposed to educational experts. And even for most politicians, the thought of putting four and five year olds into a formal school environment seems to have been unpalatable. During the late nineteenth and early twentieth centuries, the governments of 66 per cent of countries worldwide chose six as the school starting age, while in 22 per cent (including some of the most educationally successful nations) they preferred seven years old.

That leaves only 12 per cent of countries worldwide where children start school at five or younger. Interestingly, this 12 per cent consists of the four nations of the United Kingdom, and a selection of its ex-colonies and protectorates, including Australia and New Zealand.[1] In effect, every wide-eyed, wondering child around the world who starts compulsory schooling *before* the age of six is the great-great-grandson or daughter of the British Empire.

So why, back in 1870, did Victorian politicians decide to send children to school at such a young age? There's an apocryphal story that they chose five in order to go one better than Prussia, which had recently settled for six. I've never found any official confirmation of this, but it certainly accords with my own experience of educational politics: international competition and point-scoring are powerful drivers.

It *is* on the record, though, that the most important considerations in 1870 were economic ones, determined by the needs of big business rather than small children. Child labour had recently been outlawed, so elementary education was considered 'of great utility' for keeping poor children off the streets while their mothers went to

---

1   This chapter focuses on the English education system, which has inevitably influenced policy and practice in other English-speaking nations, with nods to the influence of the USA. See Appendix 2 for more information about Scotland, Wales, N. Ireland, Australia and New Zealand.

work. The early-starting age was also a sop to irate employers, who had recently been deprived of numerous cheap, biddable workers: the sooner school started, the sooner factory fodder could be released at the other end.

The early-start policy was quickly absorbed into the national consciousness. And once children were out of sight in their primary schools, they remained out of mind, so for over a hundred years what happened to them there was of little interest to politicians or the general public. Even when, in the middle years of the twentieth century, people began to ask questions about the efficacy of state schooling, solutions were always sought in changes to secondary and tertiary education. Comprehensive schools and polytechnic colleges were introduced, examinations and qualifications redesigned, universities expanded...

It wasn't until the 1980s that the political spotlight swivelled once more on to the under-elevens. By this time, Britain's heavy industry was in terminal decline and it seemed the nation's future success would depend upon 'a knowledge economy'. Secondary teachers, under attack for their students' academic performance, pointed out that the problems started in primary schools, where many children were failing to pick up the basics of reading, writing and arithmetic.

The result was fierce controversy among politicians and academics about the best way to teach the three Rs at primary level, but no one dreamt of questioning the wisdom of starting formal education so early. After a century of habit, everyone assumed that packing off five year olds to school was completely normal. Indeed, in England they were soon ready to accept an even younger starting age.

Economic considerations again. By the late 1980s working mothers were, as in Victorian times, once more the norm and the English government offered to grant free 'early years education' for four year olds – an apparent boon for both families and employers. The cheapest way to provide this education was to enrol four year olds in primary school, in the class for the youngest children, known as 'reception'. Since schools are paid per capita to educate their pupils, most primary headteachers welcomed these tiny new recruits – the policy was affectionately known in the profession as 'Bums on Seats' – and an even earlier start to education was rapidly normalised. Within a decade or so, the overwhelming majority of English four year olds were in reception classes, including 'summerborns' who'd only just celebrated their fourth birthday.

Everyone out of step but us

Why, then, did the rest of the world opt to start schooling at least one year (and up to three years) later than the Brits and their former colonies? When the fashion for state-provided education began in Europe in the nineteenth century, there was no scientific evidence on which to base the decision. There was, however, a long history of education for more privileged children – at least the male ones – which had traditionally begun around seven years old.

The historian of childhood, Hugh Cunningham, tells us that, since Roman times, European adults thought of childhood in three seven-year chunks: '*infans* up to seven, *puer* [boy] seven to fourteen, and *adolescens* from fourteen to twenty-one'. It was the *pueri* who went to school, and that tradition continued long after the Roman Empire had disintegrated. In the chivalric system of the Middle Ages, for instance, the son of a wealthy family would stay at home until the age of seven, then go to another privileged family as a page for seven years of chivalric education, before beginning another seven years' apprenticeship as squire to a knight.

This pattern is echoed in attitudes to childhood around the world. The prophet Mohammed said that 'the first seven years are for play, the second seven are for discipline and education, and the third for keeping with the adults', and according to an ancient Japanese aphorism: 'until seven years old, children are in the gods' domain'. It seems that, in terms of school starting age, worldwide ancient wisdom accords with many of today's most successful education systems.

In the nineteenth and early twentieth centuries, European

educationists such as Frederick Froebel (1782–1852), Rudolf Steiner (1861–1925) and Maria Montessori (1870–1952) developed educational programmes based on observations of children's intellectual development (see Chapter 2). They also held fast to the belief that 'the first seven years are for play', which meant that pioneers of education for the under-sevens took a different approach from schooling systems for older children. Froebel coined the term *kindergarten* (literally: children's garden) for the world's first Institute of Play and Activity for Small Children, and the schooling systems set up over a hundred years later by Steiner and Montessori (and now held in high regard around the world) also adopted an essentially play-based approach until children are seven years old.

When the science of developmental psychology began to emerge, its two earliest luminaries – Piaget in France and Vygotsky in Russia – provided scientific evidence that the first seven years or so of children's cognitive development is qualitatively different from later stages. Ever since, there has been a significant difference between the ethos of early years educational systems worldwide, and those of traditional schooling.

There are many different names for systems of early years education around the world – nursery school, pre-school, playschool – but I've chosen to use the Froebelian term 'kindergarten' throughout this book, partly because it avoids the term 'school' (see also Chapter 2). The younger children are, the more the educational emphasis has to be on helping each one *develop* various physical, emotional, social and cognitive abilities – as opposed to *teaching* skills and knowledge, as in traditional schooling systems.

The power of play

Kindergartens stress the importance of play, which is the natural means by which young human beings have always explored, experimented and developed understanding of their social and material environment. Along with adult support and guidance, children's own active, self-directed play is now widely recognised as critical to the development of:

- physical coordination and confidence, the ability to focus attention and control behaviour
- emotional strengths, including a can-do attitude, resilience and the patience to pursue long-term aims rather than immediate rewards
- social competence, such as getting along with their peers, working collaboratively in a group and communication skills (including active listening)
- cognitive capacities, such as the use of language to explore and express ideas, and a 'common-sense understanding' of the world and how it works, which underpins mathematical and scientific abilities.

To enrich and support children's own play, kindergarten education usually includes frequent opportunities for children to be outdoors in natural surroundings, and stresses the age-old (and fundamentally playful) human activities of song, dance, story-telling, art and drama. All this is combined with adult-led activities (of growing length and complexity as the kindergarten years go by), designed to lay firm foundations for children's future success at school. But developmentally based kindergarten education isn't merely about 'school readiness'. It's about readiness for life in general.

Perhaps the most significant difference between kindergarten and schooling, then, is that the former takes the 'bottom-up' approach of helping individual children develop their full potential, and the latter takes a more 'top-down' adult-directed approach involving transmission of an agreed curriculum and the expectation that all children should achieve specific educational standards deemed appropriate for their age-group. So, while kindergarten practitioners ask themselves, first and foremost, 'What is this child interested in? What support does she or he need to move forward?', the emphasis for school must be on 'What does this child need to know? What skills do I have to encourage in order to ensure she or he gets there?' A kindergarten approach to learning is often described as 'play-based' or 'child-centred', as opposed to the more formal, curriculum-centred methods employed in traditional schooling.

The great question, of course, is *when* children are ready to move from a play-based to a more formal approach, and at the heart of this debate we usually find the vexed question of literacy. Many children are clearly ready to read and write long before they're six or seven but, while kindergarten teachers would support and encourage early interest of this kind, they wouldn't want to emphasise it to the detriment of a child's overall development (that complex mix of physical, emotional, social and cognitive capacities outlined above and described in more detail in Chapters 2 and 4). They certainly wouldn't require kindergarten children to decode a reading book unless they showed an interest, or expect them to write before they were physically competent to do so. By contrast, in early-start countries *all* children are expected to reach certain goals in reading and writing at five, or even younger, regardless of their interest or their individual stage of physical development.

The unhurried attitude in countries with a later start to formal education seems to be linked to a more benign attitude to young children among the adult population in general, including concern that youngsters enjoy opportunities to play for as long as possible. When I talk to parents and teachers in other parts of the world about English children being instructed in literacy skills at four, most are horrified. I've heard several teachers describe the approach as 'cruel', while a Dutch headmaster simply laughed and said, 'Here on the mainland, we educators think you Anglo-Saxons are mad!'

The quest for the three Rs

Nevertheless, there's usually method in madness. Perhaps, back in 1870, those English politicians reckoned that the sooner children started formal education, the better they'd do in the long run? The Victorian poet Matthew Arnold, whose day job was as an inspector of schools, described the duty of elementary education as 'to obtain the greatest possible quantity of reading, writing and arithmetic for the greatest number'. He and his colleagues therefore expected instruction in the three Rs to begin as soon as children started school. Arnold was, however, right in thinking that these educational aims wouldn't be achieved by poorly qualified teachers employing punitive teaching methods to control classes of sixty or seventy pupils, which was often the case in schools serving the poorest areas of the country.

Fortunately, over the next half century conditions in UK primary schools gradually improved (teachers were better trained and class sizes decreased). Children's performance in the three Rs improved with them, and alongside rising levels of literacy and numeracy came a steady narrowing of the gap between rich and poor. Both these factors were clearly related not only to changes in schools but to improvements in diet, housing and general social conditions, including the development of the welfare state.

My own family's experience was typical: thanks to social and educational progress they moved over three generations from extreme poverty to moderate prosperity. As one of the third generation, I started school in 1953, and became – like many of the baby boomers – the first in my family to attend university. By the early 1970s, I had become a primary teacher myself, and firmly believed that all was for the best in a rapidly improving system, that universal literacy and numeracy were well within the nation's grasp and that greater equality of opportunity would follow in their wake.

Then, suddenly – and quite unexpectedly – the trend went into reverse. Despite the fact that living conditions for most British families were better than they'd ever been, the achievement gap mysteriously began to widen again, and social mobility ceased. According to UK research published in 2013, young people in the second decade of the twenty-first century are on average less literate and numerate than their counterparts fifty years ago, and also lag behind youngsters in other western countries. At the same time, social mobility in Britain has decreased significantly since the 1970s, and our country is now less socially mobile than most of the developed world.

It's desperately sad that – despite considerably higher living standards and advances in teaching methods and materials – UK schools are not delivering 'the greatest possible quantity of reading, writing and arithmetic to the greatest number.' While the reasons are undoubtedly complex, it would be amazing if aspects of primary education weren't involved. And one of the most significant differences between education half a century ago and education today is the approach to early years.

Back in the 1950s the influence of developmental psychology had stretched its tentacles even into the English educational system, and my memories of a reception class in 1953 are of dressing-up clothes, a 'home corner', sand and water play, songs, rhymes, storytime, nature walks and learning how to tie my shoelaces. The nearest we four- and five-year-old pupils came to the three Rs was 'Ten Green Bottles' and the alphabet song: serious teaching of literacy and numeracy didn't start till Year 1.

The reminiscences of other baby boomers suggest my experience is not unique. I suspect that, for a few decades after the Second World War, formal schooling for most children in England began at the same age as their European counterparts: six. At the very least, their early years at school were far less pressurised than they are for children today.

The primary wars

Part of the reason for this informality in mid-twentieth century English reception classes was the special relationship between the UK and the USA. America had unshackled itself from Britain long before the introduction of state-sponsored education, and most of its States – like the rest of the world – chose six as the age when children were admitted into the first grade of elementary school.

However, American children enter school premises at five,

because they traditionally spend a year in a kindergarten class. By the 1950s, US kindergarten practice was very much influenced by the European educationists mentioned above and amounted to a gentle, child-centred transition from home or nursery into a formal school environment. My reception experience was almost certainly influenced by fashionable trends in American education.

Unfortunately, however, these trends were soon to cause educational havoc. By the 1960s, many American educationists were convinced that this 'child-centred' approach should be extended upwards from kindergarten into elementary schools. They argued that since the key to successful learning is motivation, older children would also learn better if they learned through play. Throughout primary school, they should be supported in discovering facts and ideas for themselves, and the teacher's role should be as 'a guide on the side', not 'the sage on the stage'. These progressive theories met fierce resistance from more traditionalist thinkers, who believed in the straightforward transmission of knowledge. The debate soon became polarised and politicised, and spread around the English-speaking world.

During the 1970s and 80s, the progressive philosophy was very much in the ascendant. In England (as in some areas of the USA) it became the default model of many influential educationists, who urged primary teachers to abandon any methods seen as 'traditional'. As a primary teacher and headteacher during this period, I was by no means alone in finding these polarised views frustrating – surely the most effective teaching involved a sensitive balance between the two approaches?

We worriers were particularly concerned about the effect on literacy teaching – in their most extreme form, progressive methods amounted to giving children picture books and leaving them to work out how to read for themselves. It seemed obvious that, however motivated they were, most children would not learn to read and write a complex language like English unless they were taught something about how it works, especially phonic encoding. It was also becoming clear that the children whose progress was most affected by lack of explicit teaching were those from the poorest homes.

In my case, fate – in the form of motherhood – intervened and when I re-emerged in the 1990s as an educational writer, politicians on both sides of the Atlantic had joined the debate. They were taking increasing control of primary education and insisting on a return to more structured teaching methods. At first, many teachers were relieved at these developments, but we hadn't foreseen *how* the US and UK governments would impose their new regime, how far the pendulum would swing back, and the knock-on effects for younger and younger children.

No child left behind

By the turn of the century, educational policy in America was firmly under the control of central government, influenced by traditionalist zealots who'd won the battle about teaching methods. In 2001, George W. Bush's government passed an act called 'No Child Left Behind', requiring year-on-year improvements in reading standards and introducing a draconian system of standardised testing to keep teachers on task. Unsurprisingly, the tests were narrow in focus and based on the acquisition of specific skills that could be easily measured. Schools were also encouraged to adopt 'early intervention' programmes to prepare for this high-stakes testing, thus dragging kindergarten teachers into the target-driven fray. Indeed, ever since 'No Child Left Behind', in most states of the USA formal education has effectively begun at five, or (as parents became terrified that their child might be 'left behind') even younger.

Similar policies were being pursued in England where, in 1998, Tony Blair's government introduced National Strategies for literacy and numeracy, based on the same regime of tests, targets and – an exciting added extra for teachers on this side of the Atlantic – performance league tables for schools. These measures combined with other policies (and the spirit of the times) to ensure that the demands of high-stakes standardised testing have dominated English primary education ever since. (In fact, England now boasts the most frequently tested children in the world.)

Coincidentally, while all this was going on, concern was also growing in the UK about the hotchpotch of pre-school childcare provision springing up around the country as more and more mothers went out to work. A group of English early years experts was commissioned to create a regulatory framework called 'Birth to Three' for the care of children outside the home. Another group was asked to devise a two-year Foundation Stage Curriculum, defining 'desirable outcomes' for the education of three to five year olds. This Foundation Stage would encompass a wide range of provision, from F1 (any out-of-home care for three year olds, from nursery school to pre-school playgroups and childminders) to F2 (the primary school reception class, where most four-year-old bums were now firmly on seats).

By this time I was working as a consultant to the National Literacy Strategy, helping write their training materials, and frequently found myself attending high-powered meetings in government offices. At that time, like most of my Strategy colleagues and our political masters, I knew practically nothing about child development (or indeed what nursery and reception teachers actually *did* all day), so couldn't see why those 'desirable outcomes' shouldn't include a few literacy targets, such as phonic knowledge, a basic sight-word vocabulary and the ability to write the alphabet. It would be a great help to us in achieving our aspirational literacy goals.

I was therefore rather surprised when the early years experts resisted, arguing that such a move would be 'developmentally inappropriate' and that the emphasis before six years should instead be on children's social, emotional and spoken language development. There was one day in particular when they became positively strident and our leaders had to apply significant pressure to bring them into line. I wasn't present at that meeting but someone commented later that there were 'blood and feathers on the floor'.

However, in those days literacy specialists were a real power in the land, so our collective will prevailed and 'aspirational' literacy and numeracy targets were included in government guidelines going out to all nursery schools and reception classes. The schoolification of English pre-schools had begun. As the target-based agenda took hold, three-year-old children would soon be weeping as nursery nurses coaxed and cajoled them into trying to write their names...

More haste, more problems

Mea culpa then. You must have guessed that I have more than an academic interest in this subject. Not long after the arguments in Westminster, I became concerned about the number of children diagnosed with developmental disorders, and began research into the effects of modern culture on child development. The more I found out, the more horrified I became at the process we set in motion on the day of blood and feathers.

All the international evidence suggests that the optimal time to start formal teaching of the three Rs is around six or seven. Even though some children do learn to read easily at five, or even younger, by the time they reach double figures their average test performances are no better than those of children who start formal schooling two years later. In maths and science, there's also plenty of evidence that practical experiences and opportunities for real-life problem-solving lay better foundations than pencil and paper work. Due to the complexity of human development, the idea that 'the sooner they get started on the three Rs, the better they'll do' simply doesn't hold water.

On the other hand, there can be a heavy price to pay for children who *don't* cope with an early start. There's a growing body of international research showing that the social and emotional effects of early formal instruction can contribute to lifelong problems, affecting the health and career paths of the individuals concerned. One recent study, the Longevity Project in the USA, involved analysis of an enormous mass of data accumulated over eighty years, and concluded that starting formal schooling before the age of six is associated with 'less educational attainment, worse midlife adjustment, and most importantly, increased mortality risk'. In 2012, the chief researcher on this project wrote:

> I'm very glad that I did not push to have my own children start formal schooling at too young an age, even though they were early readers. Most children under age six need lots of time to play, and to develop social skills, and to learn to control their impulses. An overemphasis on formal classroom instruction – that is, studies instead of buddies, or 'staying in' instead of 'playing out' – can have serious effects that might not be apparent until years later.

It's not easy to prove these long-term causal links, because the consequences of too-early pressure for academic achievement obviously vary depending on children's personal biological make-up, gender, socio-economic background, and so on. Much of the longitudinal research conducted in this field relates to children from disadvantaged homes (although the Longevity Project cited above focused mainly on middle-class Californians who were 'intelligent and good learners'). Nevertheless, it's reasonable to conclude that if the effects are experienced by a large number of children in a society, they'll also impact on the wellbeing of the society itself.

While there are obviously many other variables to take into account, it's interesting to compare statistics for the UK with those for Finland, a country where children spend three or four years in kindergarten before starting formal education at age seven. The UK has less-than-inspiring scores in international comparisons of educational achievement and a shamefully low record in surveys of childhood wellbeing. It also has one of the widest gaps between rich and poor and the fourth-highest incidence of family breakdown in Europe. Finland, on the other hand, has regularly topped the European charts for literacy and numeracy, and also scores high in the childhood wellbeing stakes. It has one of the smallest gaps between rich and poor, and the lowest rate of family breakdown in Europe.

Why, oh why?

So, given the weight of the evidence, why do so many English-speaking nations remain committed to an early start? If there are no long-term educational advantages and significant long-term losses in starting school so young, why don't we just raise the school starting age and introduce a kindergarten system for younger children?

As already suggested, part of the answer must be that it's simply a national habit. And bad habits are remarkably easy to pass on through the generations. I witnessed another example of this as a young primary headteacher, when I had a couple of depressing encounters with angry old men who supported corporal punishment in schools: 'Well, I was regularly beaten,' they fumed, 'and it never did me any harm.' Fortunately, public opinion finally overruled their particular prejudice and corporal punishment was banned in UK schools in 1987. Unfortunately, most of us have never given any thought to another highly questionable aspect of schooling, handed down from Victorian times and normalised by familiarity. After all, we've been sending children to school at five for 150 years and it never did us any harm...

Recently, the downward trend towards early schoolification has been influenced by another national characteristic – one the Brits share with Anglo-Saxon nations around the world, including our cousins across the pond. We're fiercely competitive. So when international league tables for educational achievement first appeared in the early 2000s, our politicians were determined to rise higher in the listings (indeed, the Obama administration relaunched the 'No Child Left Behind' project under the title 'Race to The Top'). And, since governments have only four or five years in which to make their mark before seeking re-election, this has always been a quest for short-term results. So far – despite a signal lack of success – that's meant more and more of the same: tests and targets, resulting in top-down pressure for an ever-earlier start on formal instruction.

It's not as if educational experts haven't suggested other ways forward. Over the last three decades, many respected voices have spoken up for a less pressurised approach to the early years. In England as long ago as 1994, a report for the Royal Society of Arts led by the distinguished academic Sir Christopher Ball suggested raising the school starting age to six and providing part-time nursery education for children of three and over. Early years experts have regularly complained about the 'too much too soon' agenda ever since, and a campaign with this name has been running since 2008. In 2009, the Cambridge Review of Primary Education, organised by Professor Robin Alexander (one of the most highly-respected figures in UK educational circles) again recommended raising the school starting age, on the evidence-based grounds that an early-start regime 'dents children's confidence and risks long-term damage to their learning'.

But history leaves deep scars. The primary wars of the 1970s and 80s have left English politicians of all political colours deeply distrustful of what they call 'the educational establishment' (or, during Michael Gove's reign as Education Secretary, 'the Blob'). Fury at the misguided progressive educationists who caused such chaos three decades ago has hardened into deep-seated prejudice against any academic who doesn't wholeheartedly embrace current government plans and policies. So research studies that don't fit the policy are ignored, and critiques of the status quo – including the Cambridge Review's highly authoritative, evidence-based report – are summarily dismissed.

Long-established custom, national competitiveness, entrenched political opinions: it's a powerful cocktail. But there's a further ingredient: in countries with no real tradition of kindergarten education, there's also widespread ignorance about what developmentally appropriate education actually looks like.

Anglo-Saxon attitudes

I thought long and hard about writing 'ignorance' there, because it's such an emotive word. In the end, though, it's probably preferable to 'cruel' or 'mad' and – when knowledge about the subject isn't in the public realm – it's also understandable.

Over the last thirty years, as more and more pre-school children needed out-of-home care, private nurseries sprang up around the country so government had to assume a regulatory role. Politicians and civil servants inevitably focused their attention on aspects of care that they and the general public understood, such as health and safety, and (since the increased need for out-of-home care also coincided with the literacy and numeracy drive) the potential of out-of-home childcare for bumping up educational standards. This national lack of understanding about the way young children learn is illustrated in the most influential government document of the time – *Every Child Matters* – upon which all major policy was based. In all its 108 pages, the significance of play in learning isn't mentioned once.

These Anglo-Saxon attitudes were also compounded by the media. In 2004, for instance, at the height of my own child development research, I happened to be watching the BBC morning news programme on the day that a major report on 'highly effective' nursery schools was published. The nurseries in the study were highly effective because they adopted a developmentally appropriate kindergarten approach. But, while the BBC news commentary accurately described how high-quality pre-school practice supports early language and learning, the accompanying images didn't illustrate the sort of language activities you'd see in an effective kindergarten: songs, stories and 'sustained shared thinking' (that is, involving talk with teachers and peers) about a range of interesting experiences, outdoors as well as inside the classroom. Instead we saw library footage of tiny children wearing immaculate school uniforms, sitting at desks, clutching pencils and staring silently at something labelled 'My Word Book'. I contacted the BBC and managed to get the pictures changed, but the new version wasn't much better. I suppose one shouldn't be surprised that a *British* Broadcasting Corporation is short on images of high-quality pre-school provision.

A few years later, there was another damaging development in English pre-school policy. You may remember that, at the turn of the century, a group of experts produced a document about out-of-home childcare entitled 'Birth to Three'. This included 'developmental milestones' – average expectations for naturally occurring aspects of behaviour, such as crawling, walking and talking, which actually vary greatly between different children. But for matters of political expediency, in 2008 'Birth to Three' and the Foundation Stage were hastily cobbled together into something called the EYFS (Early Years Foundation Stage) covering the care of children from birth to five. So average developmental milestones relating to a biologically determined 'bottom-up' process were seamlessly integrated with highly specific 'top-down' educational targets for four and five year olds. So, overnight, milestones turned into targets too.

This means that, ever since 2008, a target-based 'schoolified' agenda has influenced the way all early years practitioners interact with children in pre-school settings, including childminders whose 'setting' is their own home. Whether they like it or not, they are obliged by law to help children chase arbitrary educational goals rather than supporting their natural desire to learn through play. The most recent Statutory Framework, published in 2014, includes the expectation that five-year-old children will be able to:

- read and write words and sentences, spelling phonically regular words and some common irregular words correctly;
- count, add, subtract, double and halve numbers up to twenty, and discuss weight, capacity, time, distance, money and the characteristics of two- and three-dimensional shapes (using mathematical vocabulary).

There is absolutely no reason, other than political whim, to expect five-year-old children to do any of these things. Even if some five year olds (the ones who've shown an early interest in literacy and/or numeracy) are able to achieve everything on the academic 'ticklists', that certainly doesn't mean all children *ought* to do so. Indeed introducing elements of formal learning before children are developmentally ready to cope with them is likely to be counter-productive in the long run. But many nursery managers now think that, to ensure their charges can perform satisfactorily by five, they have to start work on the three Rs when children are three, or even younger.

Political emphasis on sums and spelling at an early age influences parents' attitudes too. For most English families, the EYFS (along with various government-sponsored and commercial off-shoots) has become their major source of information on child development. Its target-driven nature encourages mums and dads to see childhood as an academic race right from the beginning. This can cause deep anxiety, leading many parents to coach their little children in literacy and numeracy skills at home. And, as adult carers increasingly focus on educational targets, play is inevitably sidelined. The irony is that play is essential for early learning and healthy development; sums and spelling aren't.

***

In 2014, the UK Early Years Forum, a coalition of national organisations concerned with young children's education and wellbeing, published a 12-point *Charter for Early Childhood*, in the hope of influencing the political manifestos for the UK general election of 2015 (see Appendix 3). Four of its twelve policy recommendations, which are based on current psychological and neuroscientific evidence about early development, stress that developmentally appropriate, play-based education should be provided for children up to the age of seven.

Predictably, the main political parties made no adjustments to their educational policies: an early-start policy, accompanied by a schoolified approach to pre-school education is still the default assumption of the English political elite, with knock-on effects on attitudes in Wales, Scotland and Northern Ireland. Indeed, the English government is at present keen to get children into school-based nurseries at two, to prepare them for a 'baseline assessment' when they're four years old.

It isn't in our children's interests, or those of the societies they inhabit, to cling on to institutions and beliefs that are likely to cause long-term damage to children's health, wellbeing and learning. Or, even worse, to adapt those institutions in ways that actually exacerbate problems. It would be more productive to look at:

- what science tells us young children need for healthy development (see Chapter 2)
- the cultural factors which now inhibit that development in a growing number of children (Chapter 3)
- the best ways to prepare children for the three Rs (Chapter 4)
- how developmentally appropriate kindergarten education can help close the gender and poverty gaps (Chapter 5)
- what early years provision looks like in our most successful European neighbour (Chapter 6).

At present, the early-start countries are in a hole. It's time to stop digging.

Chapter 2
HOW CHILDREN LEARN

How the human mind develops, why young children
learn differently from older ones and what adults
can do to help them

Learning comes naturally to human beings. Our species has a
breathtaking capacity for adaptability, experimentation, analogy,
creative thought, and has the unique ability to communicate through
language. And, unless there's something seriously amiss, every baby
is born with the potential for these human skills.

However, from the very beginning, motivation is critical to
learning. When a child's actions lead to a rewarding outcome,
he or she is motivated to repeat them, and frequent repetition
strengthens learning. The most effective reward is the one nature
has equipped human beings to enjoy – that exhilarating feeling of
personal achievement when we rise to a challenge, solve a puzzle
or get something right under our own steam. The sense of working
towards such satisfaction is known in psychological circles as
intrinsic motivation. It's far more likely to develop a lifelong love of
learning than extrinsic motivation, when the rewards are dished out
by someone else in the form of praise, smiley faces, stickers or ticks
on a test paper.

There's also the danger of motivation draining away if a child doesn't experience success very often – perhaps because there aren't enough opportunities for certain types of learning or the challenges on offer are too demanding. Lack of practice and repeated failure can both diminish children's interest in particular activities.

So how can adults help the next generation to pursue this natural learning drive, rather than losing the inborn incentive to learn? The more aware we are of our own role in the process, the better we can support children in becoming fully functioning human beings with minds of their own.

Born to learn

Birth–three
In the first few years, children need constant adult assistance on their quest to understand what's going on around them. Their first carers, usually parents and other family members, also provide models for human behaviour (including language) and support them physically and emotionally until they can explore the world on their own terms. Most of these early lessons happen without either child or parents really noticing. In their book *The Scientist in the Crib*, US psychology professor Alison Gopnik and two eminent colleagues explain it thus: 'We know a lot to begin with, we learn much more, and other people *unconsciously* teach us.' (My italics.)

Three–seven
Once they're up, running and able to communicate, children need time to develop as *independent* learners. They're primed by nature to use their newly acquired physical, social and linguistic skills to try and figure out for themselves how the world works, and their own place in it. The more opportunities they have to develop deep, 'embodied' understanding during this period, the stronger the foundations upon which later, more abstract learning will be based.

Throughout these years children are developing (and, with luck, refining through voluntary practice) the capacity to control their own behaviour, in terms of both body and mind. This is known as **self-regulation** and is essential for independent thought and action throughout life. The most helpful adult input in terms of self-regulation is sensitive support for children's own self-directed learning.

It's also possible to teach this age-group new skills that they *don't* find intrinsically motivating. Since the under-sevens are still very much at the mercy of their adult carers, they usually cooperate for the reward of approval (or avoidance of disapproval) from the grown-ups. However, this can lead to reliance on extrinsic motivation which may affect their attitude to learning in future, and perhaps diminish their ability to think for themselves. And if the skills to be taught are intellectually or physically beyond them, the emotional consequences of failure can affect their disposition to learn in the future.

Seven–adulthood

By around the age of seven, most children are sufficiently mature in terms of brain development to exercise conscious control over their thoughts and actions, meaning they're now ready to embark on increasingly complex, abstract learning tasks. Since many of the skills and knowledge required to flourish in a sophisticated twenty-first century culture (such as the three Rs of reading, writing and reckoning) require 'top-down' help, from now on teaching and learning go hand in hand. If children have had plenty of opportunities to develop as successful learners in their own right, they should be ready to soak up new knowledge and enjoy acquiring new skills, thinking creatively and working hard to overcome any problems they encounter.

This book is, of course, about the most helpful types of child-directed learning and adult support during the kindergarten years (ages three to seven), particularly in terms of developing children's powers of self-regulation and their disposition to go on learning once formal schooling begins… and indeed, beyond.

However, since development is a bottom-up process, children's needs once they reach kindergarten age depend on what's happened since conception, so I'll start with a couple of sections on two important aspects of children's learning *before* the age of three. While still involving psychological jargon like 'intrinsic motivation' and 'self-regulation', this learning process is as old as the species so is actually based in some very obvious, everyday vocabulary:

- the most important quality adult carers can bring to early learning is **love**
- and the most important ingredient children bring to the process is **play**.

Birth to three – tuning in to people

An obvious example of adults 'unconsciously' teaching their offspring is the way babies learn to talk. They're all born with the potential to speak any language on earth but, around the age of one, they start talking in their mother-tongue because that's what they've heard around them every day. Gradually, the brain cells associated with speech sounds that aren't used in their environment shrivel away, which is why it's so difficult to learn a very different language as one grows older.

Even before they're born, babies pick up the rhythms of their native tongue in the womb. After birth, they gather further data about speech sounds and language patterns when they listen to 'motherese' (the exaggerated singsong nonsense-talk that mothers tend to use by instinct) and the songs and rhymes that adult carers use to soothe and entertain them. I reckon traditional nursery rhymes have survived through the generations because they emphasise the sounds, patterns and rhythms children *need* to hear. When a baby responds delightedly to an old rhyme, mum or dad is inclined to repeat it, and frequent repetition helps establish the neural networks upon which language learning depends. To begin with, of course, children don't understand a word of it: they're just enjoying the interaction, and soaking up the linguistic data.

As time goes on, babies begin to discriminate meaningful words when loving adults chat to them about ongoing events, repeatedly tell favourite stories, share picture books time and again – and, of course, when they sing songs and rhymes and encourage the child to join in. By the end of the first year, most children have started experimenting with words themselves, and through frequent meaningful exchanges, their carers help them develop their language use. Between about eighteen months and three years, there's usually a 'language explosion', by the end of which most children are reasonably competent – and highly enthusiastic – talkers.

The underlying learning mechanism is babies' inborn talent for imitation, but the extent of a child's language learning depends on the quantity and quality of adult input. The more time adults spend interacting with babies and toddlers, the better for language learning – and the more both age-groups are likely to enjoy the interactions. This is where love comes in.

Babies are programmed to 'attach' to their adult carers, which at this stage usually means their parents, who naturally love their offspring. So when babies respond positively to parental crooning, smiles and cuddles, it makes parents feel good; and when parents give their baby lots of loving attention, the baby feels good too. The virtuous circle of mutual pleasure keeps parents singing, story-telling, conversing and chatting until their offspring start chatting back.

And it's not just talking. Language is merely one of a range of human communication skills that adults take for granted, but which are important indicators of what other people are feeling and thinking. Through their face-to-face engagement with the adults who care for them, children begin learning how to interpret expressions, gestures, voice tone and a range of other non-linguistic cues. Young children's developing ability to 'read' these cues not only supports their language acquisition but is also believed by many psychologists to be the origin of 'mind-mindedness' – the awareness that every individual (including the child him or herself) has a conscious mind.[2] Mind mindedness is a uniquely human skill that underpins our phenomenal success as a social species.

Children's social and emotional development is therefore hugely enhanced by the amount of real-life interaction they experience in their earliest years, as is their cognitive development. The developmental psychopathologist Professor Peter Hobson maintains that 'what gives us the capacity to think is the quality of a baby's exchanges with other people over the first eighteen months of life.'

As far as the babies are concerned, however, all these enjoyable experiences of cuddling, face-making, story, song and chatter aren't about social, emotional or cognitive development: they're just good fun. They and the adults are playing a fascinating social game. This is where the second four-letter word comes in. 'Play' is the word we adults use to describe what children are doing when they're having fun. Human communication skills are the intrinsically motivating results of love and play.

Birth to three – tuning in to play

There are, of course, many other important elements of human consciousness that don't involve socialising. From the very beginning, babies yearn to be independent – they want to find out about the world for themselves (and, as far as possible, to control their immediate environment) through exploration and experimentation. The drive to explore their surroundings provides the motivation to develop increasing control of their limbs and bodies. By gradually learning how to exploit reflex movements, they learn to reach, roll, grasp and so on. This developing bodily control is emotionally

---

2   Human consciousness is intensely personal – it exists within each individual mind – but it's also social because we acquire and share it through our interactions with each other.

rewarding in itself, so all parents have to do is ensure their babies have a safe space in which to experiment (and perhaps place interesting objects just a *tiny* way out of reach).

Activities of this kind may not look much like 'play'. Indeed they often look like hard work – but then, as Maria Montessori famously said, 'Play is a child's work.' As long as an activity is intrinsically motivating, it's play and the child is learning something – something that may have important long-term implications. Unfortunately, babies and toddlers are often frustrated in their quests by inadequate reach, height, dexterity, communication skills and so on. They therefore appreciate having a devoted personal assistant who cares about them enough to work out what it is they're trying to do and – when necessary – provide a helping hand. Once more, love and play go hand in hand.

Not surprisingly, the more securely attached children are to their carers, the better their overall development. And research has recently established that the most securely attached children are those whose carers are 'attuned' to their children's needs. Well-attuned adults appear to be particularly skilled at 'mind-mindedness' – they empathise with the little ones in their care, anticipating their feelings, intuiting their intentions, supporting every aspect of their attempts to play by a sort of infant mind-reading. This empathic support also includes working out when *not* to help.

I reckon the most difficult aspect of supporting children's play is working out when to chip in... and when to back off. For a loving parent watching a beloved infant trying to perform a simple task, the temptation to help (and perhaps even take over) is almost overwhelming. But babies and toddlers engrossed in play are developing a very important skill – the ability to focus attention – so adult interference is often counter-productive. They may also be acquiring problem-solving skills, figuring out cause and effect or engaged in some other important cognitive activity.

Young children at play are often acting like 'infant scientists' – observing, repeatedly experimenting, learning by trial and error.

A highly attuned adult is therefore skilled at spotting the exact moment when frustration kicks in before offering support. There are also, of course, some occasions when adults need to intervene against the child's wishes. If the task concerned is a dangerous or antisocial one, the action of a diligent personal assistant is usually to provide a suitable distraction – and plenty of cuddles should the scientist be distressed at discontinuing the experiment.

On the whole, most carers are happy when children are engaged in this sort of solitary play because it gives them a break. Their main responsibility is to ensure their infant's safety and prevent damage to any valued possessions (although, increasingly, it's also important to ensure the play is 'real', rather than virtual – see Chapter 3). But the social play described in the previous section is just as vital, so catering for young children's learning involves a sensitive balance between the two.

One activity noted by researchers as particularly helpful is chatting about what children are doing, sometimes a sort of running commentary ('What are you looking for? Oh, it's panda. You're putting panda to bed...'); sometimes, once children have begun to talk, it helps to have a conversation that expands their meaning ('*Cup.*' 'Cup? Oh, you want a drink in your cup, do you? Can you find the cup?' '*Cup.*' 'Oh well done, it's on the table. Now, what do you want to drink, milk or water?'). Children develop their language skills through genuine two-way interaction of this kind, about items and events that matter to them, so the more conversations they have, the more words and constructions they learn. And the better equipped they are to think for themselves in the future.

Now we are three

By the age of two-and-a-half most children have a fair degree of control over their bodies and have developed a reasonable command of language, so their needs in terms of learning begin to change. It's probably no coincidence that, in the past, most infants of this age would no longer have the luxury of their mother's full attention – they would almost certainly have been supplanted by a baby brother or sister. They'd therefore be passed into the care of older children from the extended family or local community, with mum available only on a part-time basis. So from now on, the normal course of social and emotional development involves getting along with other children. In an age when most children have few or no siblings, kindergarten is the obvious place to learn these skills.

There's plenty of research showing that from the age of three, pre-school education is beneficial for children, although in the early stages a few hours a day is all that's required. Some children are clearly ready for this sort of 'educare' before the age of three, but others aren't – all adult decisions about the best kind of care in the earliest years must depend on intimate knowledge of the child concerned. (Attunement again.)

Throughout *Upstart*, when referring to the most successful sort of early education system, I've used the word 'kindergarten' rather than 'nursery school' or 'pre-school' because – as described above – at this stage children still need an approach based on nurture rather than schooling. For this reason, I think it helps to avoid the word 'school', especially in early-start countries where there is ingrained confusion about what early education actually involves. Froebel's analogy of a 'children's garden' makes the point that nature still plays a significant a part in the process. But just as plants thrive best when carefully tended by skilled gardeners, children thrive best when supported by highly attuned, caring adults who understand the subtleties of human development.

Three-year-old children starting their kindergarten education are inevitably at very different stages of development. There are many possible reasons for these differences, for instance:

- development isn't a straightforward linear process, and some children naturally take longer than others to mature in terms of specific aspects of learning

- at admission some children are chronologically younger than others: at this stage, an age gap of months, or even weeks, can make a huge difference (see also the information on 'summerborns', Chapter 5 and Appendix 5)
- boys tend, on the whole, to lag behind girls in terms of language and social development, although they may be more physically confident and more inclined towards exploratory play (see also Chapter 5)
- research shows that children from disadvantaged homes often lag behind those from wealthier backgrounds, in terms of general development or, frequently, because they have less well-developed language skills (see also Chapter 5)
- a small proportion of children may suffer from a developmental condition, such as a language disorder, ADHD, dyspraxia or autistic spectrum disorder (see also Chapter 3)
- children who have enjoyed very close relationships with their carers during their first few years may be generally more advanced than others, but may find it difficult to adjust to the absence of their beloved 'personal assistant'. What's more, if their primary carer wasn't particularly well-attuned, they may be overly dependent on adult direction and thus in need of more opportunities to develop as independent learners. Unfortunately, this is increasingly the case, because (as I know from personal experience) many modern parents have been educated out of the ability to tune in to a small infant's mind.

Particularly in the early stages, then, kindergartens must offer a highly nurturing environment, in which care comes before education. 'Care' is a tricky word – it's not the same as 'love', but as far as childcare is concerned, it has to involve the sort of emotional attunement to children's needs that love inspires in a relaxed and confident parent.

As time goes on, education increasingly takes centre stage, but always on the understanding that cognitive development is interwoven with physical, emotional and social maturation and that – until children have well-developed self-regulatory powers – adult input must be carefully tailored to the appropriate developmental level. The best kindergarten staff are therefore well-attuned adults with a wide knowledge of child development.[3] And one of the most important elements of this support is, of course, providing an environment in which children can play.

The state of play

Research on the value of play in children's learning has been mounting for many decades. It is a vital ingredient in all four developmental strands (physical, emotional, social, cognitive) – some psychologists claim it's as essential to children's physical and mental health as food and sleep. Being at the heart of learning, it encourages a vast range of human strengths, such as curiosity, mental flexibility, problem-solving, self-reliance, creativity, imagination and the ability to bounce back from difficulties and learn from mistakes. It's even recognised by the United Nations as a fundamental human right of every child (Article 31 of the United Nations Convention on the Rights of the Child).[4]

However, children's play is so varied that it's almost impossible to pin it down in words. One definition widely used by playworkers is 'freely chosen, personally directed, intrinsically motivated behaviour that actively engages the child', which is quite a mouthful but accurately sums up what's involved: play is activity that is chosen by

---

3   At present in the UK, people from many different backgrounds work in early years settings, including nursery nurses, playworkers, early years teachers, and teachers who originally trained for primary education, not to mention childminders who work in their own homes. The current all-embracing terminology is 'practitioners' and, since it avoids the word 'teach', I'll use it henceforth when referring to early years staff in general.
4   Incidentally, UNICEF errs on the safe side in terms of age: it defines the 'early years' as birth to eight.

the child, controlled by the child, done for the child's own satisfaction, and involving the child's attention in an active way. When I ask adults to remember playing as kids, they usually agree the best sort of play took place outdoors (preferably out of the direct supervision of adults), was often shared with friends and didn't require any particular equipment – activities like building dens, making mixtures, inventing imaginary worlds, and so on. This is, of course, the sort of play that children have engaged in throughout the millennia, and – like the play described in the sections about development from Birth–Three – there are sound evolutionary reasons for it.

It's therefore a matter of deep concern that children's habits of play have changed almost beyond recognition over recent decades. These changes, and their developmental consequences, are discussed in Chapter 3, but the outcome is that for many children 'play' at home is now highly commercialised, devised by adults, often confused with relatively passive screen-based entertainment, and largely conducted indoors. In countries that don't have a long tradition of kindergarten education, much of the play children engage in at school and pre-school may be highly supervised for health and safety reasons or organised by practitioners to meet some educational target.

There's no doubt that playful, structured, adult-directed activities are helpful in laying sound foundations for later school-based learning – indeed, primary teachers know that, even after formal teaching has begun, the more playful a lesson is, the more children are motivated to engage and learn. But if play is to perform its developmental magic in the early years, there must also be many opportunities between the ages of three and seven for children to enjoy the time-honoured, freely chosen, child-directed activities described above. Well-attuned practitioners, like well-attuned parents, know when to back off.

The self-regulatory skills that underpin children's capacity for independent learning are hugely complex, and depend on the perennial combination of physical, emotional, social, linguistic and cognitive development. Self-regulation includes the ability to:

- identify feelings and manage emotions
- control the focus of attention and persevere with chosen tasks
- empathise with others and adapt behaviour appropriately
- monitor and reflect on one's own actions
- identify and use successful strategies
- plan ahead for increasingly complex sequences of behaviour.

Play is the means by which evolution has adapted human children to develop these skills. During the four years of kindergarten education, there is inevitably a change of emphasis from child-chosen, child-directed play to adult-directed (but still playful) activities. The timing and pace of that change varies depending on the children involved but it must be informed by each child's developing capacity for self-regulation, rather than the demands of the school curriculum or standardised tests.

As Cambridge psychologist David Whitebread points out, self-regulation is not the same as 'what might be called "compliance" or some of the narrower conceptions of "school readiness".'

The play's the thing

A key characteristic of play is that it's *active*, and thus hugely significant for physical development and self-regulatory skills. Crawling, climbing, running, jumping, skipping, sliding and generally rollicking about all contribute to children's large-scale motor control, and also to their feelings of confidence in their own bodies. Lack of opportunities for large-scale movement for three to seven year olds therefore inevitably affects emotional development. In boys, this may result in behavioural problems; in girls, it's more likely to diminish the motivation to engage in active play, and render them generally risk-averse (see also Chapter 5).

Small-scale motor control is also vital if children are eventually to be able to sit, listen, focus attention and control their behaviour in appropriate ways when they eventually reach the classroom.

Fiddling, mixing, building, cutting, sticking, painting and drawing, constructing, threading, manipulating and generally messing about with stuff all contribute to this type of control and to hand–eye coordination. Education enthusiasts tend to value and promote this sort of play (except, perhaps, the fiddling and messing about) because the long-term results are clearly of educational value, but children are likely to engage in it repeatedly only if they're intrinsically motivated to do so. Girls seem more naturally motivated to engage in small-scale play at an earlier age than boys... or maybe they're just keener to please the teacher (see Chapter 5).

When I ask adults to remember their favourite play activities, many women mention making petal perfume – an activity which seldom involves adult supervision – and laughingly concede that, although they did it lots of times, it didn't actually work till they laced it with perfume stolen from their mother's dressing table. As described earlier, frequent repetition is an essential element of play – children, acting like mini-scientists, repeatedly perform an experiment in pursuit of knowledge.

Since they've chosen the activity because they find it personally rewarding, it doesn't really matter whether the experiment succeeds or fails (either way, it's interesting). In fact, during such play, children discover for themselves that, when meeting Triumph and Disaster, it's possible to treat the two imposters just the same – a vital element of emotional resilience. They're far less likely to learn this lesson if their motivation is the reward of adult approval for successful performance of a set task.

While repetition is essential to consolidate learning, another instinctive learning strategy – imitation – is particularly relevant in social development (for instance, the shared behaviour between babies and parents described in the 'Birth–Three' sections above). Kindergarten children use 'pretend play' to imitate behaviour from the adult world: it's how they try to make sense of the vast range of human activities to which they're exposed, including trying to sort out concepts of right and wrong.

The vehicles for their role-play vary according to contemporary cultural influences – when I was a small child in the 1950s, much of our play related to the World War from which our parents' generation was still recovering; as time went on, it revolved around the battles between good and evil we saw on TV (cops and robbers, cowboys and Indians). Nowadays it's influenced by superheroes and Disney films. Whatever cultural theme children choose, pretend play also provides an excellent vehicle for exercising their own creativity and imagination in terms of costumes, scenery, props and plots. It can be as active or constrained as they choose; and there is, of course, infinite potential for the thrill of problem-solving.

Psychologists argue that role-play is a critical element in the development of self-regulatory skills. Not only do children have to work out rules for their make-believe scenario but – as actors in a play – they must exercise conscious control of behaviour. It involves countless opportunities for planning, monitoring and reflecting on their own actions. As their powers of physical and mental self-control develop, they can become absorbed in pretend play for days on end, as long as the adult world allows them the time and space to do so.

Team play

Children may, of course, engage in pretend play alone, but in a kindergarten setting it usually happens in groups, thus providing a natural vehicle for social development. Planning a scenario, negotiating rules of engagement and keeping the show on the road develops collaborative skills and a sense of personal responsibility within the group. Role play develops children's ability to put themselves into someone else's shoes, and see the world from a point of view other than their own.

Young children are naturally self-centred, so it takes time to find out how to get along with peers, deal with fall-outs, take turns and share, discover the delights and frustrations of cooperation, find out who they can and can't trust, forge friendships and maintain relationships in the hurly-burly of infant social life. In the years between three and seven, children are establishing their own sense of identity, which in a social species inevitably involves the capacity to empathise with other people, and take account of their needs and concerns. If these skills are acquired naturally through play of all kinds, they become an integral part of children's emerging personalities, which in the long-term is much better for society than unthinking conformity (or inability to conform) to social norms. The more opportunities children have to enjoy social play of all kinds, the easier they find it to see the point of socially agreed rules and to willingly abide by rules that are in the common interest.

Of course, if only for health and safety reasons, adult rules are also necessary in any kindergarten setting, but the aim is to balance these with as many opportunities as possible for children to learn social skills naturally. When things go wrong, well-attuned practitioners encourage their charges to work out a solution by talking things through, rather than leaping in to 'sort it out' for them. (One Japanese kindergarten teacher told me that her setting only had two rules: 'Don't do anything unkind and don't do anything dangerous' – plenty of openings for discussion of appropriate behaviour there.) It takes a lot of time to support children in developing social skills without intrusive supervision or direction, but the long-term social benefits are worth it.

Another way adults throughout the ages have encouraged social behaviour in their young is the use of music. Singalongs, action songs, shared music-making and dance are time-honoured ways of helping human beings to collaborate, follow prescribed rules and develop a sense of community. Another is the sharing of stories, through which the wisdom and values of one generation have, since time immemorial, been passed down to the next. Both these types of activity are as naturally attractive to pre-school children as nursery songs and bedtime stories are from birth, and an obvious vehicle for socialisation throughout the kindergarten years. (They're also vital elements in the development of children's listening and language skills, and thus for laying sound foundations for literacy and school-based learning – see Chapter 4).

The under-sevens have also traditionally engaged in rule-based activity through games like 'Here We Go Round The Mulberry Bush' and 'The Farmer's In His Den', involving rhymes and procedures handed down by one generation of children to the next. Like the old nursery rhymes, this particular aspect of childhood culture is dying out in the twenty-first century where unsupervised outdoor play is in decline. They are, however, a tried-and-tested introduction to the types of patterned behaviour required by the adult world, so kindergarten practitioners usually assume the role of older children to keep them alive. They also use age-appropriate games to introduce and/or consolidate concepts that all children need to survive and thrive as they move into the world of school.

Out to play

In the past, adults could take it for granted that children engaged in the sorts of activities described in preceding sections. Active, creative, social play – well away from grown-up interference – was normal daily activity for children of all ages. It's only in the last few decades that the younger generation hasn't been expected to go 'out to play' (see Chapter 3). So it's taken quite a while for the grown-up world to notice that what comes naturally to children when left to their own devices might be rather important for human development. Over the last few years, experts from a range of disciplines have become increasingly alarmed about this particular change in infant lifestyle. It's now clear that children who are cooped up indoors during their pre-school years will be far less likely to venture into the great outdoors as they grow older.

In 2011 – galvanised by the long-term social implications of the obesity crisis – the Chief Medical Officers for the four UK nations got together to publish *Start Active, Stay Active*, arguing the case for active outdoor play. If children haven't learned to enjoy physical exercise by the time they're seven, they'll probably be couch potatoes for life. But playing out isn't just important for physical fitness: there are mental health implications too. Spending time outdoors in natural environments has a naturally calming effect on human beings of all ages, reducing behavioural problems in schools and mental health problems throughout life.

The fact that modern children don't get out much has also attracted attention in higher education. About ten years ago, at a conference on neuroscience, I met a former mathematics lecturer who'd recorded an alarming decline in children's 'conceptual understanding' over recent years (his more everyday definition of this was 'commonsense understanding about the world and how it works' – the sensory appreciation of natural phenomena that underpins scientific and mathematical concepts). He and a colleague found, as a result of a long-term research project, that the conceptual understanding of eleven year olds in 2004 was at about the same the level as that of eight or nine year olds in 1990. When I asked him why, he informally attributed it to the decline in outdoor play.[5] Children who have climbed trees, rolled down hills, splashed through streams, made dens, forts and petal perfume tend to have a deep-seated, 'embodied' understanding of concepts like time, space, distance, and the properties of natural materials, which is very helpful if they eventually choose to become mathematicians, scientists or engineers.

There's been a further chorus of concern about the disappearance of 'free-range childhood' from business leaders and entrepreneurs like Sir John Harvey Jones, who've recognised the contribution of outdoor play to the development of problem-solving, resilience and risk-management skills. (My favourite story is from Richard Branson, whose mum apparently used to take him out in the car when he was two or three years old, drop him off a mile or so from home and

5   He also pointed out that '1990 was the year the National Curriculum moved into English primary schools, and the sand and water moved out of infant classrooms.'

leave him to find his way back. Perhaps a little early for such a serious challenge, but he reckons it worked for him.)

And there's also rising concern about the decline of outdoor play among environmentalists and natural historians who know that if children don't get out and about in the natural world, they're unlikely to develop any sort of emotional connection with nature. The embodied understanding that underpins cognitive concepts also underpins our feelings about the world we inhabit. In the words of David Attenborough, 'No one will protect what they don't care about; and no one will care about what they have never experienced.'

As the Jesuits put it several centuries ago: 'Give me a child till he is seven years old and I will give you the man.' The way young children spend their time has long-term implications for their physical and mental health, their future careers and their attitudes to the world in general. It therefore also has profound implications for society and, indeed, the planet. Kindergarten education is about preparing the next generation for life, not merely for formal schooling. And outdoor play – the birthright of all human children since time immemorial – is a hugely significant factor in this preparation. In the words of the Scottish early years pioneer, Margaret McMillan: 'The best classroom and the richest cupboard are roofed only by the sky.'

Great minds think alike

McMillan (1860–1931), one of the founders of the nursery school movement in Britain, was committed to the idea of play-based learning for children up to the age of seven and (as the quote above suggests) particularly interested in the power of outdoor play. Like Susan Isaacs (1885–1948), another UK-based expert who suggested that nursery teachers should think of children as research-workers (and themselves as observers), McMillan's name isn't well known outside early years circles. There are, however, a few international figures whose contributions are widely recognised even in early-start countries like the UK.

Frederich Froebel (1762–1842), a German pedagogue who studied under the famous educator Pestalozzi, was one of the first teachers to develop a theory of early learning. He set up an Institute of Play and Activity for Small Children and coined the term 'kindergarten'. As well as free play, the activities on offer included singing, dancing, gardening and playing with toys, known as Froebel's Gifts, which he'd devised to develop children's natural learning potential. Some of today's educational toys, such as building blocks of different geometric shapes, are based on Froebel's insights.

The next well-known figure in early education was **Rudolf Steiner** (1861–1935). He was an Austrian polymath whose interests included philosophy, social reform, alternative medicine, spirituality, art, architecture, dance and education. He founded the Waldorf School in Germany, with a kindergarten stage for children between three and seven. Steiner believed that during the first seven years of life, children are influenced by 'the will' and learn best by imitation. His kindergarten emphasised the development of empathy, connection with the natural world, music, the arts and participation in a range of practical activities. There are now around two thousand Waldorf kindergartens worldwide but Steiner's opinions on human spirituality were controversial, which has sadly had an impact on broader acceptance of his educational legacy.

Maria Montessori (1870–1952) was an Italian doctor who devised a range of teaching methods and materials for mentally disabled children. These helped them make remarkable progress and, as a result, Montessori was able to develop a scientific theory of early education, based on observation of children in the school she founded for two to seven year olds (*Casa de Bambini* – literally 'Children's House'). Her methods include practical activities, freedom of movement within the classroom and outdoors, and (voluntary) use of teaching equipment designed to support naturally developing skills. She also insisted on child-sized chairs, tables and so on, to help develop her pupils' independent use of materials. Her philosophy has spread worldwide, resulting in many thousands of dedicated Montessori schools, and many more that use some Montessori methods.

Jean Piaget (1896–1980) was the Swiss psychologist who first charted developmental stages, starting with the 'sensori-motor stage' (birth to two) and the 'pre-operational stage' (two to around seven). He showed that learning at each stage builds on what has gone before, and emphasised the importance of practical, 'concrete' activities for young children. He introduced the idea of developmental 'readiness', suggesting that top-down teaching will be unsuccessful if a child isn't ready to learn. Although his work is now contested in certain respects, it was highly influential in English-speaking nations during the mid to late twentieth century, and his 'schema' theory about the acquisition of knowledge has similarities with the neuronal networks described by modern neuroscientists.

Lev Vygotsky (1896–1934) was born in the same year as Piaget. He was a Russian psychologist whose work was suppressed by the Soviet regime and was thus not widely known until the 1980s. However, he is now acknowledged as a major figure in developmental psychology for theories stressing the role of social interaction in learning. These include:

- the significance of symbolic systems ('cultural tools'), especially language and the way it shapes human thought
- the sensitive support of children's learning by more experienced mentors, at times when they're trying to do something that's just beyond their current capacity (on such occasions the child is said to be in the 'Zone of Proximal Development' or ZPD).

He too believed that seven was the appropriate age for more formal schooling and that a young child engaged in self-directed play is, in developmental terms, 'a head higher than himself'.

In the zone

Since the rediscovery of Vygotsky's writings, there's been debate over two significant differences between his developmental theories and those of Piaget:

- Piaget claimed children's grasp of a concept comes *before* they use language to explain it, while Vygotsky believed that language precedes and aids conceptualisation.
- Piaget argued that children must be developmentally 'ready' to learn for themselves; Vygotsky claimed that, when in the ZPD, they can be supported in taking the next step forward.

The idea of the ZPD has been extremely influential over recent decades and has sometimes been used (wrongly) to justify explicit, formal, top-down teaching of young children. In fact, Vygotsky and Piaget both argued that children 'construct' their understanding of the world on the basis of their interactions with it. A child's ZPD is, therefore, specific to his or her developmental stage and circumstances, and adults must take account of that in terms of the support they provide. The American psychologist Jerome Bruner talks about 'scaffolding the learning' in the ZPD, rather than teaching, and it's often a matter of tailoring the circumstances in some way to make a task more achievable. The mother who, for instance, places a toy *just* out of her baby's reach is successfully scaffolding his learning when, with a little effort, he can achieve his goal and experience the pleasure of success.

According to Vygotsky the most effective support is aimed towards the higher level of the child's ZPD – the edge of challenge. If mum places the toy too close, there's less pleasure involved when the baby grasps it because the goal has been too easily gained; if she places it too far away, he may fail to reach it and thus experience frustration. Judging a young child's ZPD therefore requires a high level of attunement on the part of adult scaffolders.

This has profound implications for kindergarten practitioners. Not only must they understand the basic principles of child development, but they must also be highly attuned to the individual children in their care, at a developmental stage when levels of understanding, language and self-regulation vary widely. And in the later kindergarten years, practitioners have to bear in mind the specific skills and abilities their charges will need during the next stage of education and help them – whatever stage of development they're at – to move gradually (with the aid of intrinsic motivation) towards 'school-readiness'.

Unfortunately – especially in countries with an early school starting age – working with pre-school children isn't regarded as a high-status profession. Since looking after small children has, along with other domestic tasks, traditionally been thought of as 'women's work', it's also low paid. Most parents and politicians see childcare up to the age of five as little more than babysitting, so don't consider practitioners' qualifications particularly important. Once schooling begins at the age of five, early years primary teachers, while at least recognised as professionals, are expected first and foremost to *teach,* rather than to support children's development.

The principal aim of this book is to develop public awareness of the kindergarten stage (three–seven) as critically important for the next generation's long-term wellbeing and educational success. If it's recognised as such, the qualifications and professionalism of those who care for children in the early years are clearly of considerable significance. The widespread practice of using minimally qualified staff and requiring them to follow a simplistic, centrally prescribed framework is simply not good enough.

Many of the pre-school practitioners I meet in England are highly attuned, caring individuals who are deeply concerned about the potential damage they're doing by pushing children towards academic learning too early. But their lack of professional qualifications means they're not confident enough to challenge the 'educational' targets of the EYFS. And since nursery managers are usually under pressure from anxious parents and primary schools for children to be 'school-ready', staff are urged to tick as many of the EYFS's 'educational' boxes as early as possible. In 2012, the Nutbrown Review of early education and childcare qualifications made many sensible suggestions for improving the professionalism of the workforce. But while the review was officially 'accepted' by the government, its recommendations were largely ignored.

The UK does in fact have a very proud tradition in terms of early childhood education (as do other early-start countries) but it's always been the Cinderella of the educational system and the expertise of highly qualified early years specialists is seldom acknowledged or respected, even in educational circles. As the dismissive 'blood and feathers' comment illustrates (see section 'No child left behind' in Chapter 1), 'nursery teachers' are at the very bottom of the academic pecking order. And once schooling starts at five, the only ZPDs most primary teachers have time to take an interest in are those they hope will help drive children through the next set of tests.

I think it's fair to say that, in terms of understanding what the under-sevens *really* need from the educational system, most politicians in early-start countries haven't even entered their own Zone of Proximal Development. So there's a lot of work to be done to ensure the UK has a highly qualified early years workforce, one in which professional understanding *and* human attunement are valued and rewarded.

Everything to play for

'Give me a child till he is seven years old, and I will give you the man.' This quotation, attributed to St Ignatius Loyola, the founder of the Jesuit Brotherhood, actually refers to the effectiveness of early indoctrination, in his case into the Catholic faith (and the truth behind it is now exploited daily by marketers bent on achieving brand allegiance in society's youngest consumers). Indoctrination was not, however, the aim of the great minds cited in the two preceding sections. Their interest was in the nurturing of human understanding, creativity and   motivation to learn during the stage of development when 'the imagination is warm and the impressions are permanent'. And they all recognised that it takes around seven years of enlightened adult support for young human beings to develop the self-regulatory skills that make them successful lifelong learners.

There are also, of course, sound humanitarian reasons for giving young children space and time to enjoy and learn from play before enrolling them in formal schooling, especially now that – as will be described in the next chapter – there are so few opportunities for *freely chosen, personally directed, intrinsically motivated activity that actively engages the child*. A carefree childhood is a gift in itself, and play is a major source of childhood wellbeing.

Nevertheless, in early-start countries, there's still great suspicion about the efficacy of play-based education, particularly in political circles. Politicians still remember the Primary Wars waged in the latter decades of the twentieth century when 'progressive' educationists took developmental principles to extremes and many primary-aged children were denied the explicit teaching they needed to become literate and numerate. The inevitable political backlash helps explain the English-speaking world's current obsession with 'school readiness'.

Upstart's argument is that seven is the age at which every 'great mind' has agreed that the majority of children are as 'ready' as possible to benefit from a more 'top-down' approach to learning. And, as pointed out in Chapter 1, a dedicated kindergarten stage doesn't mean holding them back if they show an interest in any aspect of the three Rs. Indeed, as will be illustrated in Chapters 4 and 6, in an environment that supports and celebrates literacy, most children *want* to read for themselves well before they reach their seventh birthday and, with sensitive individual support, can usually develop the skills needed for reading fluency. Similarly, when play involves numbers and calculation, children *want* to learn numeracy skills and record their thoughts with symbols.

With plenty of time for sensitive Vygotskyan scaffolding of the tasks involved, most children will make good progress. But simply forcing them to undertake complex cognitive challenges before they're mentally and physically mature enough to meet them is counter-productive in the extreme. Even those children who show early interest in the sorts of academic learning valued by adults need time to acquire the physical competence and confidence, emotional resilience and social skills underpinning self-regulation. In an educational culture where 'success' is measured merely in terms of test results, it's easy to forget that the capacity for independent learning involves a great deal more than passing exams, and that the ways children learn in their early years will impact on every aspect of their future lives, health and wellbeing.

This was widely understood in previous generations, when precocity was generally frowned upon and children were expected to behave like children. (As an early reader, I remember my grandmother's regular cry of: 'Our Sue, you've always got your head stuck in a book. Get out and play with the other kids or you'll go funny.') But in a period of rapid social and cultural change, we've become used to hearing that 'children grow up more quickly these days' and intellectual precocity is often valued at the expense of physical, social and emotional aspects of development.

In evolutionary terms, this is a serious backwards step. As US developmental psychologist Alison Gopnik points out:

> If you look across the animal kingdom, you'll find that the more flexible the adult is, the longer that animal has had to be immature. I think that even the term pre-schooler is a bit misleading. It implies that our job is to get children ready for school and that school is where the important things happen. But pre-school isn't just about readiness. It's an important stage in its own right.

***

I began this chapter by emphasising the importance of two key ingredients for young children's health and wellbeing – love and play – and the significance of adult 'attunement'. Nowadays, most children can't bank on the availability of full-time parental love for more than a year or so; thereafter, they generally rely on care outside the home – so it's increasingly vital that their carers are highly attuned adults with a sound understanding of child development. Young children's need to be loved and cared for is in direct conflict with their similarly intense drive to explore and experiment for themselves, so it takes talent, knowledge and commitment on behalf of kindergarten practitioners to work out when to intervene in their play and when to back off.

I've also stressed the significance of *time* for the under-sevens to learn through play. The next chapter argues that – in an age of screen-based, competitive consumerism – children's play has been hijacked by commercial forces in ways that can seriously undermine their capacity for self-regulation. The state education system is probably the only means of countering this assault on early childhood. Introducing a ring-fenced kindergarten stage for three to seven year olds – staffed by caring, well-qualified practitioners – is a way of reinstating play in all children's lives.

Not only would this allow children a few carefree years in which to enjoy their childhood, it would also give them a much better chance of growing up bright, balanced and with minds of their own.

Chapter 3

TWENTY-FIRST-CENTURY CHILDHOOD

How modern life can damage healthy development...
and how a play-based kindergarten stage could help
put things right

In spring 2014, a young mother arrived for the Open Day of an expensive pre-prep school in the south-west of England. She proudly told the teacher how good her three-year-old son was on his iPad, and a demonstration revealed that he was indeed a wonder – a truly talented techno-kid. However, the nursery staff soon noticed that in other respects the little boy's development was not so wonderful. His balance was poor; although he could walk, he often preferred to crawl; and his spoken language was around the level expected of a child half his age.

Gradually, the mum noticed the difference between her son's behaviour and that of the other children visiting the nursery. 'She went very quiet and next time we looked they'd disappeared,' the nursery teacher told me. 'She was Asian and perhaps she was isolated from the rest of the community. She probably hadn't mixed much with other mums and children so she'd had no one to compare him with.'

The special needs explosion

I heard this story on the day it happened, at a talk I was giving about my book *Toxic Childhood*, which I was revising at the time for a new edition. It was a disturbing reminder of why I'd researched and written a book about modern childhood in the first place. It's also what finally convinced me to do everything I could to spread the word about the significance of 'real play' in the early years of children's lives.

As a literacy specialist, I certainly didn't expect to spend fifteen years of my life researching child development and end up championing play-based learning. It happened because, around the turn of the century, I was travelling round the UK giving talks about phonics, spelling and grammar and thus meeting thousands of primary teachers every year. It didn't take long to notice that, everywhere I went, teachers were worried about the children in their classes.

There was, they told me, an explosion in the numbers with 'special educational needs' (SEN), especially developmental disorders, such as attention deficit hyperactivity disorder (ADHD), dyslexia, dyspraxia (problems with physical coordination) and autistic spectrum disorder (ASD). But this was merely the tip of the iceberg. My notebooks from the time are filled with comments about widespread changes in the behaviour of children who didn't have any diagnosable special needs. I lost count of the number of times teachers reported 'poorer listening skills', difficulty in 'getting them to attend', an increase in 'low-level behavioural problems' and children 'not getting along with each other as well as they used to'.

The chorus of concern was louder in disadvantaged areas of the country, where I also regularly heard the refrain 'language is going down year on year' (see also Chapter 5) but teachers in the leafy suburbs were similarly worried. It seemed that – according to the people who worked with them every day – children *in general* were finding it more difficult to focus their attention, control their behaviour and cope with the social give-and-take of classroom and playground.

When I checked out the SEN statistics, I found there had indeed been a huge increase in developmental disorders over recent decades. Dyslexia, which had first reached public attention in the late 1970s, was now widely recognised and could often be ameliorated by intensive teaching support, but it was still causing real problems for about 10 per cent of children. ADHD, which didn't even exist as a 'condition' until the early 1980s also now affected about one in ten children in the USA and UK. The increases in ASD were even more alarming: in the USA in the early 1980s it apparently affected only one in 50,000 children; by 2004 this had rocketed to one in 166 (when I checked again in 2015, it was 1 in 68), and again, the UK situation seemed to be similar. I couldn't find figures for dyspraxia, the new kid on the special needs block, which I'd first heard about in the mid-90s, but according to SEN specialists it was increasingly widespread.

Psychologists agree that there's an inborn neurological predisposition to all these conditions, and the 'explosion' has often been put down to improvements in diagnosis – as researchers become more aware of the characteristics of specific learning difficulties, it's easier to label children's problems. But, during my time in education, the increases had been so dramatic that I'd always thought there must be something else behind them.

The reason these life-changing problems are called developmental disorders is that they all relate to human abilities that are expected to develop 'naturally' over the course of early childhood (and which we therefore take for granted) – abilities associated with aspects of what I've now learned to call self-regulation. All those teachers' comments about children's behaviour *in general* made me wonder whether aspects of modern children's lifestyles could sometimes be causing predispositions to developmental disorder to kick in harder? And whether the same factors were affecting the behaviour of more and more children who couldn't be described as having 'special educational needs', but were just finding it a little more difficult to focus their attention, control their behaviour and 'get along with each other'.

The thought was a scary one, with implications not only for each and every twenty-first-century child, but for the way we care for and educate them, and for the society they'll eventually inherit. So it seemed worth finding out which features of modern life might be implicated and whether there was anything we could do about it.

How special is special?

It took eight years to research and write *Toxic Childhood* because it involved interviews with scores of experts from a wide range of disciplines, each of whom pointed to complex inter-relationships between many contributing factors. I found myself investigating all sorts of things: diet, sleep habits, exercise and play patterns; changes in family life (particularly opportunities for communication), parenting styles, childcare and education; and the impact of consumer culture and technological progress on child development as a whole.

Not surprisingly, I soon came to the conclusion that the subject is immensely complicated. There are 'toxic' elements in every one of my research areas, and most of them overlap with several others. What's more, our culture now changes so rapidly that damaging habits of behaviour often become embedded in our daily lives before anyone spots that they might be harmful. There is, however, no doubt that, over the last few decades, some aspects of childhood have changed beyond recognition – and all of these are linked to the development of attention, physical coordination and/or social skills.

Soon after the book was first published in 2006, there was a further flood of research showing that those turn-of-the-century teachers were right to be worried about their pupils. For instance, in the same year, UNICEF gave the USA and UK rock-bottom ranking in a survey of childhood wellbeing (20th and 21st out of 21 countries in the developed world). Considering that, at the time, these two nations were ranked first and fourth in terms of economic prosperity, such a poor showing was both staggering and shameful.

In the UK, as well as rocketing SEN statistics, a 2006 national study found that at least 50 per cent of children from disadvantaged areas were arriving at school with significant language delay (see also Chapter 4) and a couple of years later a survey in one English local authority found 80 per cent of new entrants were less well physically coordinated than children in the past. There have been similar findings in the USA, along with a longitudinal study recording a downturn in levels of empathy among college students over the last thirty years, with a particularly steep drop since the turn of the century (by 2010, 75 per cent of students scored lower than their peers of thirty years ago).

Government reports on various aspects of childhood have also flowed thick and fast since 2006, but government responses have so far been decidedly half-hearted. They generally amount to declarations of concern and occasional 'sticking plaster' solutions, designed to deal with specific issues. There's so far been no coherent attempt to tackle toxic childhood syndrome as a whole. Meanwhile, changes in children's behaviour are increasingly being 'normalised' – we seem, as a culture, to be accepting a general deterioration in aspects of development as inevitable.

This was graphically illustrated in England in 2010, when the definition of special educational needs was revised at the instigation of Ofsted (the Office for Standards in Education). Over the preceding seven years the number of children whose problems were assessed as severe enough to merit extra educational help had increased from 14 per cent to 18 per cent of the school population – if this trend continued, by 2020 a quarter of the nation's children would be labelled 'special'. Providing specialised extra help for so many school pupils would of course be prohibitively expensive, so Ofsted decided that around half the children diagnosed with special needs (essentially, those with comparatively low-level developmental disorders) simply needed better teaching and more pastoral support. In other words, the phenomenon of mushrooming problems with aspects of self-regulation has been accepted, and quietly normalised, by the political and educational establishment.

But it certainly hasn't gone away.

I ❤ my iPad

Let's get back to the three-year-old iPad enthusiast. Was his physical and linguistic immaturity due to nature or nurture? The gaggle of early years teachers with whom I discussed the question that evening decided it was probably a mixture of both. But we also agreed that if the little lad *hadn't* spent so much time on his iPad, and his first three years had instead been filled with experiences like those described in 'Birth–three' in Chapter 2, his problems with movement and language wouldn't be anywhere near so bad. Within a year, neuroscientists in the USA released the first research backing up our suspicions: the excessive use of tablet computers by the under-twos can adversely affect their overall development.

When I was writing the first edition of *Toxic Childhood,* iPads were merely a gleam in Steve Jobs's eye – indeed, until their launch in late 2010, the market for tablet devices was pretty small. Since then, they've become a must-have addition to the average home's battery of screen-based equipment, taking their place alongside TVs, laptops, smartphones and console games. In the words of US psychologist Daniel Anderson:

> As a society, we are engaged in a vast and uncontrolled experiment with our infants and toddlers, plunging them into home environments saturated with electronic media. We should try to understand what we are doing and what are the consequences. [6]

---

6   Like me, Anderson had previously worked as a consultant for children's educational TV – until the TV companies started aiming programmes at the under-threes.

The trouble is that all these electronic devices were originally invented for adults, not children. From an adult point of view, they've generally been an enormous boon, providing a range of short-cuts to communication, information and entertainment that previous generations couldn't even begin to imagine. And since this is the world our children are born to inherit, as each new device came on the market, there didn't at first seem any reason to deny them access to its many delights.

But it's steadily become clear that there's no short-cut to healthy child development and learning. Today's children may be growing up in the twenty-first century but they're still born with the same brains and bodies as their Stone Age ancestors – biological evolution is a long, slow process. Throughout human history, it's taken around two decades for each generation to develop the physical, emotional, social, and cognitive skills they need as adults, and that fact doesn't change just because the culture changes. Indeed, modern neuroscience also shows that it still takes twenty-odd years for the brain to reach full maturity and that the early years of children's lives are particularly critical in its development.

Today's children are in particular need of self-regulation skills because it takes considerable self-discipline for human beings to remain in control of technological devices, rather than letting the technological devices control them. On an over-populated planet, they'll also need empathy and social skills to ensure that they can get along with each other, not only in day-to-day contact, but at a global level.

It's already been shown in Chapter 2 that play in the early years is a vital factor in the development of all of these human abilities. And while children are born primed to play, they don't automatically know that some things might be dangerous to play with – this is, of course, why parents put child-proof locks on kitchen cupboards and keep little children away from fires and cookers. Since screen-based entertainment didn't appear to be dangerous – and it's taking many years to assemble the research proving that it is – marketers have developed products to cater for ever-younger age-groups.

Handheld devices have proved particularly attractive to babies and toddlers (not least because mum and dad spend so much time gazing at them). By 2014 tablet-ownership had spread to over 70 per cent of UK households, and of the pre-schoolers in these families, a third actually have their own tablet. App-based games are popular among the under-ones because you don't need to be able to walk and talk in order to enjoy them. And it hasn't taken long for busy parents to discover that smart phones and tablets make great 'pacifiers', wonderful for keeping little children busy while adults attend to other tasks. It's very easy in these circumstances for a small child to become hooked on screen-based fun, and once that's happened it's difficult for mum or dad to take this particular pacifier away. There's even a joky term for the fuss they kick up when you try: it's called an 'iPaddy'.

Over the last five years, therefore, sedentary screen-based entertainment has steadily become the default activity of many babies and toddlers, despite advice from the American Academy of Pediatrics that children under two should have *no* screen time at all. It is, however, a rare parent who follows this advice – or, indeed, the AAP's recommendation for children over two, which is no more than one to two hours' recreational screen time a day. The average in the UK is currently around five to six hours.

Junk food and junk play

Normalisation of damaging and potentially addictive behaviour isn't new, of course, and neither is public reluctance to follow medical advice. For instance, over the course of the twentieth century, technological advances in food production led to massive increases in consumption of 'junk food' – tasty, time-saving meals and snacks that provide little actual nourishment but an awful lot of calories and additives. Nutritionists became concerned about the long-term effects of feeding this stuff to children as long ago as the early 1970s, but their warnings went largely unheeded until the turn of the century, when a worldwide obesity crisis forced everyone to wake up to the problem.

The nutritional message is now gradually getting through: it isn't just 'junk' as in rubbish, but 'junk' as in *junkies*. When young children develop a taste for food that's been carefully designed in laboratories to stimulate their tastebuds, it's extremely difficult to wean them off it. The World Health Organisation now recognises obesity as one of the most serious global public health challenges of the twenty-first century, so the human race has certainly learned this lesson the hard way.

The good news in the UK is that a combination of public information campaigns, educational initiatives and market regulation is gradually making an impact – by 2015 the obesity rate in children under ten appeared to be levelling off. The bad news is that it took forty-five years for the adult world to recognise and act upon the recognition that technology-driven lifestyle changes can seriously affect children's physical and mental health – even though, over that period, we actually *saw* them growing fatter and unhealthier.

The even worse news is that, in the same way that the global food industry transformed children's eating habits, their habits of play have been transformed by the growth of global toy, fashion and entertainment industries. Once upon a time, play was something children invented for themselves when left to their own devices – as described in Chapter 2 it's a *natural* process (*freely chosen, personally directed, intrinsically motivated behaviour that actively engages the child*). Nowadays, however, we automatically associate it with manufactured products, usually something children have seen on a screen, such as TV and film tie-ins, princess and superhero paraphernalia, and various much-hyped highly advertised toys of the moment. From a developmental point of view, most of this stuff is rubbish – and it's also highly addictive. So the time has come to flag up the analogy between junk food and 'junk play'.

Screen-based entertainment, for instance, combines continual high-level sensory stimulation with minimum physical effort –

exactly the opposite sort of activity from the time-honoured 'real play' through which human children develop resilience and self-regulatory skills. There's also precious little personal effort involved in other sorts of play bought in the shops – usually the main reward is the immediate thrill of acquisition (just watch a child at Christmas, immediately tossing aside one highly desired present so as to get on with unwrapping the next). This means that the younger children are when junk play becomes their default activity, the less effort they'll be willing to expend on real play as time goes by. In fact, junk play has also made a significant contribution to the obesity crisis – once it's become a substitute for the real thing, children are far less active, so burn off far fewer calories.

There are, of course, profound implications in the growth of junk play for children's learning and wellbeing. By short-cutting to quick-fix fun, they miss out on the repeated, exploratory, experimental activities that underpin physical, emotional and cognitive development. And when they get their kicks from screen-based entertainment, they also miss out on opportunities to develop the linguistic and social skills that come from first-hand, real-life interaction.

Consumerism, concern and control

Both junk food and junk play are products of a global consumer culture, but while junk food is to some extent coming under regulatory control, junk play is flourishing as never before. In economic terms, there's a simple reason for this: there'll always be a market for food. In the long run it doesn't matter to global corporations if some parents choose to reject junk and feed their children fresh produce (or, at least, products that limit ingredients found to be damaging) – the market can provide whatever the punters want, as long as they're prepared to pay for it. In a global economy, there's no way twenty-first-century citizens will resort to self-sufficiency by growing their own food.

But real play costs little or nothing in monetary terms – indeed, it actually relies on children being self-sufficient and growing their own. It's also far less subject to parental control than food because the role of responsible adults is often to back off and let children get on with it. So there's no role for consumerism in the provision of real, healthy play – how could a global corporation ever sell parents something that's so resoundingly *free*?

There *is*, however, plenty of money to be made by encouraging parental concern about their offsprings' present and future wellbeing. Ask any parent what they want for their children and the response will inevitably involve words like 'safe', 'happy' and 'successful'. So the market has invented a whole new branch of consumerism – the parenting industry – through which to target mums and dads who are beginning to recognise the dangers of junk. It caters for twenty-first-century parents' lack of time for spending with their offspring (and often their lack of confidence about how to spend it), coupled with anxiety that, in traffic-choked urban environments, children can no longer just go out and play with their chums as they did in the past.

There are now therefore innumerable 'fun' products on the market, designed to keep children occupied and out of harm's way, while simultaneously maximising their learning potential. The most obvious are screen-based games claiming to hone various cognitive and visual-motor skills, which appeal to modern mums and dads keen to prepare their children for a digital future.[7] To cater for physical development, some of these gadgets are designed to get youngsters dancing, exercising or just swooping about the house or garden. For parents who'd prefer their offspring to learn in a less constrained and remotely controlled environment, there is another way to throw money at the play problem – children's

---

7   Many of these are labelled 'educational', although this word has disappeared from products aimed at children under two because there's enough scientific evidence to suggest a connection between these products, ADHD and language delay.

clubs and classes offering activities that tick various boxes on a 'developmental' wish-list.

There's no doubt that many of these clubs and classes can be valuable, or that many of the people who devise and supply them are genuinely motivated to enrich children's lives. But any pre-packaged activity, chosen by adults to enhance children's chances of success, is inevitably a 'top-down' substitute for the 'bottom-up' experience of real play. This, by its very nature, must originate in the children themselves and proceed with minimal interference from the grown-up world. Though supervision is necessary for safety purposes, it should be with the lightest possible touch.

It's only when they're free from top-down control that children can begin to realise their own identity, creativity, learning potential and capacity to think for themselves. Even young children need this freedom, because without frequent opportunities for self-directed play, how will they ever learn to control the focus of their *own* attention, regulate their *own* behaviour and get along with peers under their *own* steam? Yet, from the moment they're born, the lives of most twenty-first-century children are tightly controlled from morning to night – filled by adults, if not with mindless junk, then with 'worthwhile' adult-controlled vehicles for top-down learning.

It's not as if parents are universally happy about the change in children's recreational habits. On my travels round the UK, I meet many who'd love to let their offspring 'out to play' in the time-honoured way, but who still feel obliged to buy into commodified alternatives. Quite apart from fears about traffic, they explain that a pre-teenaged child outdoors without adult supervision is now such a rare sight that they don't want their son or daughter to be 'the only one'. Not only would there be no one else around to play with, but unsupervised young children now stand out like a sore thumb, putting them at increased risk from 'stranger danger'. So parents who let their children play in the local neighbourhood are often labelled 'irresponsible'.

This constant surveillance of children has rapidly become normalised, and the freedom to play in ways favoured by human evolution has virtually disappeared from many young lives. We've reached the stage when, in the words of naturalist Stephen Moss, 'Britain's children in some ways have less freedom than free-range chickens.'

Normalisation, nature and culture

It's surely no coincidence that the steady disappearance of real play has happened alongside a steady increase in developmental delay and disorder. While a multitude of lifestyle factors contribute to 'toxic childhood', the two key drivers of healthy development have always been parental love and children's freedom to play. Both have now been comprehensively hijacked by screen-based competitive consumerism.

There's fierce competition by global brands to 'own' children from the earliest possible age, with the result that most children now learn, often even before they can talk, to equate both love and play with stuff they see on-screen and in the shops. Parents, as the gate-keepers to the next generation's minds, are also influenced by market forces into confusing love with a toxic cocktail of indulgence (because pester power is extremely difficult to resist) and control (because who wants to be thought irresponsible?). Even though many parents are uncomfortably aware of this process they feel powerless to resist, as these quotes from a 2011 UK government report on the commercialisation of childhood indicate:

> It's crept up on us gradually and makes it difficult to make a stand.

> We have all become so used to the ubiquity of these images and messages that we no longer always register them constantly.

> It's the cacophony of advertising messages everywhere that make it hard to escape.

One mum who'd attempted to register a complaint against a marketing campaign summed it up: 'I felt that I was a small fish in a big ocean swimming against the tide.'

We seem to have reached a point when anyone who questions the value system behind the corporate takeover of childhood is considered a 'grumpy old person', hideously out of touch or just plain weird. But the many challenges confronting humanity in the twenty-first century won't be solved by repeating the mantra 'It's the economy, stupid.' Parental love arguably is the most important emotion in our species' repertoire so attempts to pervert this love for financial gain are against the most fundamental of human values. Similarly, when cultural norms deflect children from activities that are vital to their healthy all-round development, something is fundamentally amiss with the culture.

The last decade or so has seen the emergence of a number of campaigns challenging the commercialisation of childhood. But the charities behind them – such as the Campaign for a Commercial-Free Childhood in the USA and the UK's Save Childhood Movement and Bye Buy Childhood – exist on a shoestring, so they're unlikely to make much impact in a global consumerist culture. A professor of social marketing recently compared their efforts to 'wandering round the trenches during the First World War, handing out leaflets on how to avoid the bullets.' If parents are to be supported in resisting commercial assaults on their emotions and rallied in the cause of real play, they need more powerful allies against consumerism.

In some countries, national governments have stepped in to help. Sweden, for instance, has banned marketing to the under-twelves and France has banned terrestrial broadcasting to under-threes. Although it's virtually impossible to police these restrictions in a global marketplace, they at least make it clear to parents that commercialisation and screen-time are not in children's best interests.

Until the UN starts to take a stronger interest in these issues, perhaps the most productive way for national governments to inform and support parents is via universal medical, educational and children's services. In some countries, such as Finland, this is already the case, but in the USA and UK the current approach is usually to wait till things have gone very wrong, then offer mum and dad the chance to attend 'parenting classes'.

The perils of modern parenting

When writing *Toxic Childhood*, I kept putting off the chapter on parenting, due to a mixture of guilt, suspicion and fear. Guilt because, as a late-twentieth-century parent, I'd been a typical modern mum and felt awful about all the junk food my daughter had consumed and the many hours she'd spent in front of a shining screen. Suspicion because, from a professional point of view, I had growing misgivings about the contribution of the parenting industry to 'helicopter parenting' (mum or dad constantly hovering over their offspring). And fear because I was frankly terrified at the sheer quantity of research material piling up in a corner of the office. So, when finally obliged to wade through it, I was delighted to find it boiled down to a simple message that seemed both sensible and (given that parents know the basics of child development) reasonably achievable.

There's one well-documented parenting style that psychologists in western societies widely acknowledge to be effective. It's usually called 'authoritative parenting' and involves a sensitive balance of warmth and firmness:

- on the one hand, warm, responsive, loving attention, including respect for children's feelings and opinions
- on the other, the setting of firm boundaries for behaviour at various ages, on the grounds that parents want the best for their children in the long-term, even if it sometimes causes short-term frustration.

Over time, children internalise their parents' warmth in the form of self-worth and self-confidence, and they also internalise the ability to abide by parental boundaries in the form of self-control and self-discipline. (Mind you, according to another mountain of research, this internalisation process depends on their regular access to 'real play', which doesn't always seem to be on the radar of parenting experts.)

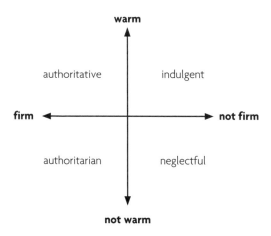

The other three styles that appear regularly in the research are far less likely to produce well-balanced children. Authoritarian parenting, where parents are firm but not particularly warm, often produces children who lack self-esteem and initiative, and who may go off the rails when the controlling parental hand is finally removed during the teenage years. Indulgent parenting (warm but not firm) can turn out narcissistic, selfish youngsters who lack the self-discipline to avoid temptation, so may also go off the rails as they grow older. And the offspring of neglectful parenting (neither warm nor firm) often end up as dysfunctional as the families that raise them.

It's easy to see how several decades of hyper-consumerism has normalised an indulgent parenting style – to the extent that it's now often considered an indication of love to 'spoil' one's child – while simultaneously persuading more responsible parents to exercise increasing control over every aspect of their children's lives. In this latter respect, commercial forces have a powerful ally in the competitive high-pressure education systems of early-start countries, which ratchet up parental anxiety about children's future success. The net result is that the next generation's freedom to develop self-confidence, self-discipline and innumerable other personal qualities and skills through real play has practically disappeared.

The more I've learned about all this, the sorrier I feel for modern parents, trying to pick their way through a child-rearing minefield far scarier than anything I encountered when raising my own daughter. How are they expected to maintain a balance between warmth and firmness in a world where love is so easily perverted into conspicuous consumption? How can they ensure the right sort of play when 'responsible parenting' has become a synonym for constant surveillance and control? In short, how can society ensure that the developmental significance of real play is as widely recognized as that of real food?

Detoxing childhood

I've now had almost two decades to ponder this question, during which I've been involved in many campaigns about different aspects of 'toxic childhood syndrome'. I've also had time to wonder why these issues seem worse in the UK and USA than other wealthy western nations, and to travel widely in Europe looking at child-rearing methods there. I've concluded that a key factor is public attitudes to early childhood, which is inevitably affected by a nation's approach to pre-school education.

A play-based kindergarten stage, such as those in the Nordic countries, normalises real play. It sends out a message to everyone

– parents, politicians, the general public – that young children need to be treated as active, creative, social individuals who are perfectly capable of learning and thinking for themselves, rather than sitting at home consuming junk or chasing adult-defined targets at school. This message has knock-on effects down into the pre-kindergarten years, because parents are less likely to be conned by harmful commercial messages. And it makes it easier for school-age children to enjoy a more free-range existence, because outdoor activities soon become widely recognized as important to everyone's mental and physical wellbeing.

It also provides a model for parents of an authoritative approach to child-rearing, in which 'warmth' translates as adult attunement, and 'firmness' as the establishment of behavioural boundaries that help children take growing responsibility for their own safety, happiness and success. I'm always impressed, in northern European countries, by how competent and responsible school-age children seem in comparison to their UK peers in all sorts of day-to-day behaviour, such as looking after their possessions, helping with domestic chores or getting around their local area by foot, bike or public transport.

That's why I'm now convinced that the best way to detoxify childhood – at least in the short term – is to give all children the opportunity for three (or preferably four) years of developmentally appropriate kindergarten education. In traditionally early-start nations like England, this would involve a massive paradigm shift. But if the politicians who run the educational show were to look for reasons behind the rising tide of developmental delay and disorders, rather than simply accepting them as inevitable, they might see how raising the school starting age is much more likely to raise national standards in the three Rs than an ever-earlier focus on schoolified learning. At present, children with developmental issues – and even those who are just a little less mature than the rest – struggle to keep up with all the tests and targets even before they cross the school threshold (see Chapter 5), thus dragging down average scores.

A 'too much too soon' approach to education is, therefore, a significant contributory factor to toxic childhood syndrome as a whole. Indeed, we've now reached the stage when – between commercialisation and schoolification – the sorts of play that young children have enjoyed since time immemorial are being squeezed out of existence. By reinstating this play at the heart of early childhood, we could give every child the time and space to develop physical coordination and confidence, emotional strength and resilience, social and communication skills, and the cognitive capacities that underpin meaningful learning and understanding.

***

In 2015, a UK government report found that 20 per cent of children between five and sixteen were now being diagnosed with an emotional, behavioural or mental health problem of some kind, including – despite Ofsted's definition-juggling five years earlier – many developmental disorders. The report was commissioned because the Child and Adolescent Mental Health Service (CAMHS) appeared to be reaching breaking point. (As one educational psychologist told me at the time, 'My clinical colleagues are overwhelmed with referrals – basically, they're doling out medication just to get kids out of the office.') Since it also found that 28 per cent of *pre*-school children now face problems likely to impact on psychological development, the situation is likely to get worse rather than better.

The government's response to these findings was to allocate more money to CAMHS – presumably so they can medicate more distressed and/or disaffected youngsters as the numbers continue to swell. Yet pathologising a steadily growing number of children and young people is neither economically viable nor fundamentally humane. On the other hand, the introduction of a kindergarten stage would:

- free children from the twin pressures of 'school and cool' at the most formative stage of their lives
- give time to sort out any problems that do arise before formal schooling begins
- provide parents with a trusted source of informed advice about child development, in the heart of every community
- help change national attitudes to early childhood.

It's not just parents and children who would benefit from such a change. Children are the citizens of the future, so all responsible adults have a vested interest in their long-term wellbeing. The following three chapters show how trusting in young children's remarkable ability to learn through play, and providing developmentally appropriate support during the early years of education, is the best way to ensure the future success and happiness of the greatest possible number. Not least in terms of providing the firmest possible foundations for literacy and numeracy.

Chapter 4
THE THREE Rs

Why literacy and numeracy are still the bedrock of
education, how children acquire the underpinning skills
and why early schoolification is counter-productive

'Look, love,' the elderly teacher said kindly. 'You people at the
National Literacy Strategy have got it all the wrong way round.
Children can't write till they can talk. They can't talk till they can
listen. And they can't bloody listen!'

It was Yorkshire, 1998, and I was speaking at a conference about
teaching writing in primary schools. If I hadn't been travelling round
the country for several years, I'd probably have shrugged off her
words as a neat variation on 'the younger generation is going to the
dogs' (as uttered by the older generation since time immemorial).
But this lady had just summed up, very succinctly, what I was
hearing everywhere, and I sought her out later for more information.
A teacher for forty years and obviously devoted to the eleven-year-
old children in her care, she'd first noticed a general deterioration
in attention skills in the early nineties and reckoned they'd gone
steadily downhill ever since. 'They're still good kids,' she said, 'but
they're all over the place compared with children ten years ago. So
it's harder for them to settle down for reading and writing.'

Tuning in to language

It was this meeting that finally propelled me on to the research trail. A couple of months later I was interviewing Dr Sally Ward, a speech and language therapist who'd found that, between 1984 and 1998, the discriminative listening skills of nine-month-old infants in inner-city Manchester had nose-dived. She explained that, unless children learn to focus on their carer's voice in very early infancy (see 'Birth to three – tuning in to people' in Chapter 2), there's a serious chance they'll suffer from language delay, with a long-term knock-on effect on learning, literacy and behaviour.

The capacity to tune in to language is the most fundamental of attention skills, one that we take for granted children will acquire naturally, particularly in wealthy countries where we can expect their basic material needs to be met. But Sally had come to believe we can't take it for granted any more: 'I don't think it's down to just one thing,' she said, when I asked what might be behind the problem. 'It's lots of things coming together.'

She listed a few – increasing traffic noise; pushchairs facing outwards so child and parent can't see each other to communicate; all-day TV distracting mums from interacting with their babies or toddlers; videos being used as electronic babysitters. We agreed that the arrival of children's channels in the early 90s – thanks to cable and satellite TV – meant parents spent less time talking and singing with their offspring.

I soon discovered many other speech and language therapists with similar concerns. One of them, Clare Mills, had managed to persuade her TV producer husband to make a documentary (*Too Much Too Young*) for the Channel 4 *Dispatches* series, pointing out the problems and contrasting UK early years practice with that in European countries such as Belgium, Switzerland and Hungary. They sent copies of it on DVD to every MP, but no one took any notice. Another, Dr Ann Locke, told me how a project she was working on in Yorkshire to improve disadvantaged children's language skills was being stymied by the introduction of the National Literacy Strategy. So it came as no surprise some years later when a survey by the speech and language charity ICAN found that at least half the children in the UK's disadvantaged areas were now starting school with significant language delay.

However, by this time, I'd also met experts from other fields who attributed problems with attention skills to a decline in physical activity. They explained that children's freedom to move around was increasingly constrained at all ages due to parental fears about safety, both indoors and out. How could they settle down to schoolwork if they hadn't developed bodily coordination and control?

Other child development experts were concerned about social skills. They told me that 'de-centring' in order to focus on what other people are saying is a social skill that some children take quite a while to acquire. So they need plenty of opportunities for social play (first with adult carers, then with peers) before they're ready for school.

As a literacy specialist, I hadn't previously paid much attention to what happens *before* children begin learning to read and write. Like everyone else, I just assumed that, unless they had specific hearing or speech problems, they'd be able to speak and listen by the time they were five. And now, dozens of experts were telling me that in a rapidly changing world, you can't 'just assume' anything about child development.

Laying the foundations

Despite my growing interest in child development as a whole, I've never lost my primary commitment to ensuring that all children have access to the three Rs. Even in a digital age, these skills are still the bedrock of education: indeed, their very acquisition reorganises the internal wiring of the human brain in ways that lead to more rational, reflective, analytical thought. While love and play develop children's human potential, literacy and numeracy make them more civilised.

Learning to read, write and do written calculations doesn't come naturally in the way that earlier learning does. As recent additions to the human repertoire, they aren't part of our genetic make-up. Instead, they 'piggyback' on natural abilities, including:

- auditory, visual and spatial perception
- spoken language
- categorisation, patterning and problem-solving skills
- various sorts of memory (auditory, visual, spatial, embodied; short- and long-term).

Each R requires children to develop and rally this wide range of natural human abilities and adapt them in highly specific ways. It can take many years of conscious effort and practice before any R becomes automatic but the long-term rewards are considerable – both for individual learners and for the society they live in.

It's not particularly sensible, therefore, to embark on such an important learning journey before children are in conscious control of their minds and bodies, and thus likely to make steady all-round progress. Some children who seem 'ready' in terms of one R, may be less secure in others – or in the social, emotional or physical maturity required to flourish in a classroom. And the progress of every child is affected if teachers are continually distracted by problems with less fortunate classmates. There's also the danger that 'well-brought-up' children will seek to please their teacher by performing set tasks by rote, without actually understanding the underpinning concepts.

This is why the vast majority of countries worldwide have chosen to start formal schooling when children are six or seven. In terms of self-regulation, facility with language and motivation to learn, allowing more time for play-based education pays dividends in the long run. Three or four years of kindergarten education also gives all children time to familiarise themselves with letters and numbers through play, while their adult carers demonstrate the manifold advantages of being able to read, write and reckon.

It's like building a house. The foundations of any building are out of sight and thus out of mind, but if they're shaky the eventual construction will always be fragile. So it's worth devoting plenty of time to getting the foundations right. Now that cultural forces are undermining the natural course of many children's development, it's more important than ever that children's formal education has a firm grounding in the natural learning drive known as play. It can, however, be difficult to argue this case with adults who have spent their entire lives believing that play is just 'messing about' and education should 'naturally' start at the age of four or five.

Anglo-Saxon attitudes versus Finnish foundations

When I tell UK teachers and parents that Finnish children aren't expected to read, write and do written sums until they're seven, many are initially appalled.

'But I was reading when I was four!'

'My daughter would be bored to tears if she were held back.'

'What do the teachers do all day if the children are just playing?'

So I've learned to follow up quickly with the following information:

- Finnish children are *not* held back – as it happens, most children do start reading, writing and doing simple calculations before they start primary school and are supported in their efforts by kindergarten practitioners, just as they would be by parents in a loving, literate family home.

- Despite the emphasis on play, there are plenty of activities led by the teacher, starting with very short simple sessions for the three year olds, and growing steadily longer and more specific as children grow older. Some of these activities hone in on skills that underpin the three Rs, some on other aspects of development, but they're all almost entirely *oral* (no written exercises or sums), so listening skills and spoken language are constantly emphasised and developed.

When I first visited Finland ten years ago, I was particularly struck by children's motivation and attention span. So was a group of Ofsted inspectors who'd visited the previous year. They commented that six year olds 'appeared to be more readily interested, to show enthusiasm or delight more frequently and spontaneously, and to have a higher boredom threshold than their English peers'. They also reported that classrooms were less noisy and the teachers were 'not preoccupied with discipline and control' as is so often the case in England.

When written worksheets are off-limits, kindergarten practitioners need to know quite a bit about the language and attention skills that underpin effective learning. Many of the short teaching sessions for the youngest children (and the teacher-led games they played) are designed with these concepts in mind. For instance, I watched a Finnish kindergarten teacher tiptoe around her setting, conspiratorially selecting four delighted three year olds to accompany her to a corner where some chairs were set in a circle.

'Here's our sentence for today,' she announced when they were all sitting comfortably, 'My name is Agneta.'[8] Each child then repeated the sentence, substituting his or her own name. It took about a minute.

'Oh very good!' she exclaimed. 'You say your sentences so well!' And the children returned to their play. I discovered later that the last time they'd played that game there had been three children in the

---

8   Agneta spoke in Finnish – I had an interpreter!

group, and that next time there'd be five. If any had found it taxing, they'd be given lots of opportunities to practise in a smaller group until ready to move on. By the time they were six, Agneta expected all children to be able to concentrate on oral activities in a large group for half an hour or so at a time. (It also occurred to me that no one would ever have to teach them what 'a sentence' is because they'd been saying them for three years.)

Contrast that with a 'circle time' for six year olds I watched a few months later in a UK school – thirty-odd children were sitting on the floor, wriggling and flopping all over the place. The teacher wasted a lot of time shushing the wrigglers and it wasn't long before everyone was bored by the activity. Tragically, these children were already in their second year of formal schooling so their personal educational building projects were based on the shakiest of language and listening foundations.

Let's hear it for story and song!

There are two extremely helpful activities, threaded throughout the day in most European kindergartens, which children enjoy enormously, and which human adults have unconsciously used to develop children's language and listening skills since time immemorial – **story** and **song**. Unfortunately, in English pre-schools and early primary classrooms there's little time to devote to them because of the need to crack on with more formal learning – after all, there's a demanding national test in phonic knowledge when children are six, and the first SATs in literacy and numeracy a year later.

Let's start with the developmental advantages of singing. Along with dancing and moving to music, it prepares the ground for phonics by developing auditory discrimination, helps sensitise children to rhythm and pattern, develops their coordination and control (including the ability to articulate clearly), and enhances connectivity between the left and right hemispheres of the brain. Singing is also very helpful for developing memory skills, upon which a great deal of human learning depends. All sorts of facts are easier to remember when set to music (the alphabet, for instance, and numbers: 'One, two, three, four, five; once I caught a fish alive!') and learning any song by heart helps strengthen children's auditory memory – that is, the ability to remember increasingly long sequences of sound. This is vital for a species that communicates in the long sequences of sound known as language.

It also explains why children enjoy songs, rhymes and musical activities so much. Nature has programmed them to do so. Evolutionary biologists believe that, even before *homo sapiens* developed language, Neanderthal parents were crooning to their offspring and yodelling messages across the hunting grounds. And anthropologists tell us that every human culture that's ever existed appears to have had a tradition of song and dance. So when an activity that aids learning comes so naturally to young human beings, it makes sense to encourage it. ('Why do you do so much music?' I casually asked Agneta. 'Music trains the mind to pattern and the ears to sound,' she replied, clearly amazed that any educator would ask such a daft question.)

Nature has also programmed children to enjoy stories. Listening to a well-told tale tunes them into the rhythms and cadences of speech and the more often an adult retells the tale, the more meaningful particular words and phrases become. The young listener thus finds it progressively easier to follow the thread of a narrative, understand the meaning of new words and expressions, and reproduce these words and phrases in their own speech. When we *read* stories to children we also develop their auditory memory for the rhythms, patterns and devices of written English so that – once they've got phonics sorted – they'll find it easy to follow the flow of written sentences, then paragraphs, then complete narratives.

Stories are important for thinking skills too. Repeated exposure to spoken narrative develops children's capacity for linear, sequential thought – the sort of thought required for logical analysis (it's no coincidence that we talk about being able to 'think *straight*'). And since the actions of the characters in stories have consequences, narrative helps drive home the significance of cause and effect, not to mention offering insights into human behaviour and opportunities to ponder moral dilemmas. What's more, while they're listening to a story, children have to 'make the pictures inside their heads', a serious contribution to their long-term capacity for mental imagery and creativity.

There are wider implications too. The educational philosopher Kieran Egan maintains that *homo sapiens* is 'a storying animal; we make sense of things commonly in story-form; ours is largely a story-shaped world' and that stories are basically '[mental] tools for organising our emotions'. Since one of the most significant factors in early childhood is learning to understand and control emotions, this gives listening to stories an important role in self-regulation as a whole.

Evolution is a remarkable process, and it's a foolish culture that throws away the opportunity for children to benefit from it. So please forgive a short return to the theme of 'toxic childhood' which, as a tribute to the importance of stories, I'll embed in an anecdote.

The little boy who said 'Fish'

About a decade ago, a fellow literacy specialist called Pie Corbett conducted a small-scale study in primary schools. He wanted to teach children some stories by heart, with the aim of developing all the cognitive processes described above. His project began with an initial assessment, which involved interviewing three children in each school – one who was considered 'able' by the reception teacher, one of middling ability and a third who was generally struggling. When he asked 'Can you tell me a story?' the results were remarkably consistent.

'Almost every time,' Pie said, 'the able child came up with a reasonably coherent story – Goldilocks or something. But the others – zilch!' Some apparently stuttered a few disjointed words and phrases, a couple sang 'Bob the Builder' and one, rather inscrutably, kept saying 'Fish'. Pie eventually found that this little lad was trying to tell his favourite bedtime story, which was *Finding Nemo*. Apparently, he watched it every night on his DVD player.

Most children's experience of stories these days involves visual, rather than auditory, processing. The boy who said 'Fish' had presumably never heard a spoken narrative for his favourite story ('Once upon a time, there was a little fish called Nemo who had a wonky fin. One morning, his daddy took him to school to meet the other fish... etc, etc') so how could he tell it to someone else? Even though he'd apparently watched it dozens of times.

But watching stories on a screen doesn't just rob children of the means to retell them. It also denies them opportunities for all the complex mental processing described in the previous section. A visual 'narrative' involves a welter of fast-moving images, music and sound effects, all of which are highly stimulating but not particularly helpful in terms of developing linear sequential – and consequential – thought. Indeed, young viewers may not even be aware there's a narrative at all. The professor of neuroscience Susan Greenfield calls screen-based experiences of this kind 'Yuk and Wow' experiences, exciting at a sensory level but with minimal worthwhile cognitive gains, like the 'junk play' described in Chapter 3.

Several years after the little boy said 'Fish', Pie and I were reminiscing about his project. 'You know how I said the able children could always tell me a story?' he said. 'Well, I got it the wrong way round. It isn't that able children can tell stories. It's that children become 'able' when someone reads them stories, over and over again.'

Nature versus culture

So to return to my earlier argument, children's increasing capacity to think in logical, analytic, reflective ways isn't merely a by-product of recently developed cultural tools, such as written language or digital technology. It depends upon sensitive shaping, within each generation's heads, of the many natural abilities that allowed *homo sapiens* to create those cultural tools in the first place.

And if evolution has programmed young children to enjoy play because it develops their self-regulatory skills, songs and rhymes because they tune minds to pattern and ears to sound, and stories because they make human beings generally 'cleverer', it's only sensible to allow time for twenty-first-century children to reap the benefits of these natural vehicles for learning. Especially when so many other aspects of their physical, emotional and social development are also enhanced by the time and space to engage actively in the 'intrinsically motivated, self-directed activities' that lucky children have enjoyed for countless millennia.

Unfortunately, the more amazing cultural tools we devise, the more difficult we find it to trust in old-fashioned human nature. Technology now provides us with so many convenient short-cuts that we're inclined to look for quick fixes in every aspect of our lives. At present, politicians in early-start countries are convinced that there are simple short-cuts to cognitive development – ways in which pre-school practitioners can accelerate children's 'school readiness' by honing some of the highly specific sub-skills of the three Rs. They believe that, rather than waste time while nature works its ancient magic, it's possible to cut to the educational chase in terms of literacy and numeracy.

The most obvious example of this is an obsession with early systematic phonics teaching. Phonics is the system by which the speech sounds of a language are represented by written letters, and combinations of letters. Linguists describe English as a 'deep' language because its phonic system is highly complex (see Appendix 4) and there are many irregularly spelled words. To anyone who spends more time with computers than small children, it probably seems perfectly logical that the sooner you start teaching human beings this complicated system, the sooner they'll be able to decode and encode words in order to read and write.

But human beings aren't machines to be programmed in a logical linear fashion – we're still the same bundles of flesh, blood and emotion that we've always been. Indeed, part of education's remit in civilised societies is to support children in learning to control those emotions. Treating them like machines may lead to some short-term cognitive gains, but it won't help turn them into well-rounded human beings who can think for themselves.

When I've tried to argue this case with English politicians and other phonics zealots, they often cite the fact that English is a 'deep' language as the reason for making an early start on systematic teaching – there are so many sound-symbol correspondences to learn that children *must* crack on with it as early as possible. Finnish, they point out, is a 'shallow' language so its phonic code is easy to crack.

They're also unimpressed by my reply that Finnish may be phonically regular but it's grammatically fiendish (for instance, it has seventeen different case endings for nouns) resulting in many long words that children must learn to syllabify correctly in order to read even the simplest text. Their kindergarten teachers nevertheless manage to cover everything the under-sevens need to know through oral activities – using games, rhymes, songs, silly stories, multi-sensory materials and carefully planned teaching sessions like the one I saw Agneta deliver. They then support children individually in their intrinsically motivated efforts to read and write... and their children are doing much better in the long run than those in England.

I've also tried to point out that, from a developmental point of view, the more difficult something is to learn, the more sense it makes to leave it till children are capable of abstract thought, such as the mental manipulation of a highly abstract system. Phonics involves the auditory discrimination of discrete speech sounds (of which most people aren't consciously aware), and then linking them to a visual symbolic code, which in English is extremely demanding (check out the intricacies in Appendix 4).

Unfortunately, these arguments have always fallen on deaf ears –

indeed, one politician actually covered his ears with his hands, like a small child avoiding unwelcome information.

Huckt on fonix

The subject of phonics inspires strong emotions. People tend either to love it or hate it (which accounts for over a century of squabbling about its importance among literacy experts). I suspect the reason is that phonics is an extremely 'left-brain' business, so anyone who has difficulty in balancing left and right brain activity would find it emotionally arousing.[9]

As a long-time fan of phonics and spelling, I've written lots of textbooks on the subject and, when it was out of fashion in the 1980s, argued passionately that most children need explicit teaching, if not for reading then definitely for writing. But, being well aware of the difficulties in both teaching and learning the phonic code, I'm firmly of the opinion that – especially in the early stages – a light touch pays dividends. Once children are familiar with the alphabet, the lucky ones (i.e. those who are good at spotting patterns, both auditory and visual, and who have also been read to regularly for many years) tend to pick up basic phonic rules pretty easily. If they also have well-developed spoken language skills and good auditory memory, they're soon able to combine phonic decoding with comprehension of written texts and go on to become enthusiastic readers.

The best sort of preparation for literacy, then, must be to ensure that as many children as possible are 'lucky'. As well as providing daily song and story-reading sessions, early years practitioners can use tried-and-tested activities, devised by early years experts through

---

9   While there's considerable debate and much utter nonsense talked about 'left- and right-brain thinking' there are undoubtedly differences between the mental processes that go on in the two hemispheres. For anyone who wants to read up on the science, I suggest *The Master and His Emissary: The divided brain and the making of the Western world* by Iain McGilchrist (Yale University Press, 2009)

the years, to develop the relevant skills (many of these activities are also relevant for numeracy, in which pattern-recognition and auditory memory is just as critical – see the section titled 'The Third R', below). In England at present, however, obsessive political focus on phonics means that a 'light touch' approach is practically impossible.

Six year olds are now required to sit a demanding standardised phonic test, including not just real words but invented ones like *foid*, *yewn* and *harnd*, so the focus in terms of literacy is firmly on decoding, while meaning and motivation fade into the background. Many nurseries take this job very seriously because they know how anxious parents are about the test (one nursery nurse told me bitterly about the time she'd wasted organising a 'phonics table' for the two year olds – 'I mean, most of them can't even talk, let alone work out what *curtain*, *caterpillar* and *carrot* have in common!').

Over-focus on any aspect of learning in the early years is riven with long-term dangers. In terms of phonics, there's a serious danger that children trained to decode without sufficient attention to other aspects of literacy learning will become as hooked on phonics (and test-passing) as the politicians who think they've found a magic bullet to solve all the nation's educational woes. The chances of their going on to become committed readers are then very small.

In 2014, the English Minister for Schools triumphantly announced that the number of children passing the Year 1 phonics test had risen from 58% to 74% over two years. He claimed this meant '102,000 more six year olds reading more effectively than would have been the case without this government's focus on phonics.' I, on the other hand, claim it means that hundreds of thousands of children under the age of six are now being systematically trained to pass a demanding high-stakes test of questionable value, with no consideration of the short- and long-term effects on their mental wellbeing or their attitude to schooling, literacy and learning.

As I said, the subject of phonics inspires strong emotions.

More haste, less success

Academics have advanced many cogent arguments against England's current policy on the teaching of reading, but from *Upstart's* point of view, Dr Margaret Clark's analysis of children's performance in the Year 1 phonics test results has particular resonance. There was one significant fact that she actually had to use the Freedom of Information Act to acquire: the older children are when they take the test, the better their performance. Well, what d'you know?

Her discovery accords with other evidence on age-related academic achievement in early-start countries, which the current government either hasn't read or prefers not to mention. For instance, a recent study in New Zealand compared children who started formal literacy instruction at the age of five with others (in state-funded Steiner schools) who didn't start learning to read and write till they were seven – by the age of eleven there was no difference in reading ability between the two groups. However, the children who started at five developed less positive attitudes to reading, and showed poorer comprehension skills than those who started later. Other studies have also shown that short-term gains from early formal instruction tend to disappear over time, but that emotional responses to the experience linger on (see also the section 'A tale of dwindling achievement' in Chapter 5).

Yet again, educational research tells us that 'too much too soon' doesn't make long-term sense. A great many four- and five-year-old children simply aren't mature enough to sit quietly while earnest adults initiate them into the intellectual intricacies of literacy and numeracy – and even those who are able to sit still may benefit more from other activities (see Chapters 5 and 6). I remember a sad little anecdote from an NLS review, during a period when reception children were expected to sit in the 'literacy corner' for an hour every day while their teacher covered the requisite targets. According to the researcher, most were bored to tears. 'It wastes your time, sitting on the mat,' one little boy confided to her. 'It wastes your life,' his chum chimed in dolefully. Bored, demotivated children don't learn efficiently and neither do those who are simply trying to please the teacher, rather than genuinely engaging with a learning task.

More time for physical development pays dividends too. There's long-standing European research evidence that some children are physically competent to write letters and numbers easily at five, most when they're six, and some aren't ready till they're seven. This certainly accords with my own experience of young children's writing progress, and that of occupational therapists called in to deal with the worst fall-out of an early start on written work. It's common for many UK pupils – especially boys (see Chapter 5) – to have difficulty in forming and remembering the shapes and orientation of some letters and numbers and many also lack the small-scale motor control and muscular development required to manipulate a pencil. Forcing them to do this before they're old enough to cope just makes the complex business of learning to write much, much harder.

On the other hand, as practitioners in European kindergartens find, children who are given time to mature – and provided along the way with activities to develop skills that make sense to them – are usually enthusiastic about recording their ideas. They're intrinsically motivated to read, write and jot down numbers like the grown-ups, so they learn to do so without pain.

The third R

Maths is not my forte so I've dreaded writing this section. I'm a perfect example of someone whose introduction to numeracy was built on shaky foundations so, although I've managed to pass all necessary exams and get by on a day-to-day basis, I lack the confidence that comes from deep-seated understanding of the principles involved. When someone asks me an off-the-cuff question requiring mental arithmetic, I panic blindly – even though in a stress-free situation with access to pen and paper I can usually rally my hard-learned cognitive strategies and work out the answer.

Unfortunately, emotional memories are much deeper-seated than cognitive strategies so, like many other British adults, I've spent my life firmly convinced that I'm rubbish at maths.

There is, however, no reason for anyone to be rubbish at maths if their introduction to the subject is based on sound developmental principles. In the early stages, some of these principles are similar to those underpinning literacy skills. Numbers, like letters, are abstract symbols – 'tools of the mind' to be manipulated according to certain long-established rules. And auditory memory is, of course, essential for counting and other memorisation tasks, such as learning multiplication tables. However, the third R soon parts company from the first two. Maths requires children to think and remember in ways that are very different from the linear processing strategies required to decode written language.

For instance, it's one thing for a young child to recognise a numerical symbol such as 7 but quite another to understand what 'seven' actually means (i.e. what exactly it is that seven stars, seven letters and seven years have in common). And although auditory memory skills enable children to reel off the numbers from one to ten, that's not the same as understanding what counting is *for*, or how it links to simple calculation. This involves visual, spatial and problem-solving skills which, as usual, are best developed over time through real life experiences.

Active, creative play (especially outdoor play) provides the 'concrete experiences' that underpin deep, embodied understanding of quantity, shape, volume, weight and so on. The mental assimilation of mathematical concepts depends on this deep-seated physical understanding. Do you remember my description in Chapter 2 of the maths lecturer who, between 1990 and 2004, recorded a serious decline in children's 'commonsense understanding of the world and how it works'? And his suggestion that this was due to two things: the decline of outdoor play and the disappearance of sand and water trays from reception classrooms?

(Ever since the global economic crisis in 2008, I've wondered whether the brilliant young men on Wall Street might have spotted the fundamental flaw in continually slicing up sub-prime mortgages if – during their early childhood – they'd switched off their computer games and got out more.)

Play also provides countless opportunities for children to engage with mathematical problem-solving, since it throws up questions like: 'How many?' 'How big/small/wide/heavy?' 'What shape/size/distance/angle?' It also provides them with opportunities to employ their dawning appreciation of number, shape, area and volume in a meaningful context. When they encounter such questions as part of their own self-chosen play, children are highly motivated to work out solutions for themselves. They benefit immensely from solving simple mathematical problems of this type without adult help. Indeed, given plenty of time to apply their inborn capacity for pattern-recognition to meaningful real-life situations, most children can work out the underpinning principles of addition, subtraction, multiplication and division – even though they're not consciously aware of doing so or of the mathematical vocabulary adults use to describe them.

It takes several years of play-based experiences to develop this sort of deep conceptual understanding, but in the long run it's time well spent. Through *talking* with their adult carers about how they personally solve particular problems, children can gradually bring their unconscious knowledge to the surface, so that when they're introduced to the language of maths in school it makes sense to them and they feel confident of their own ability to tackle mathematical problems. This approach is much more likely to produce confident mathematicians than the system by which I was taught, which involved memorising certain procedures known as 'adding', 'subtracting' and so on, then obediently completing pages of sums, to be rewarded with ticks when I got them right or punished with crosses when I didn't.

Maths, motivation and meaning

As pointed out in Chapter 2, three-year-old children vary greatly in terms of their overall development and these maturational differences can't be expected to even out till they're around six or seven. Even though children from loving, literate homes may seem ready to make a start on the three Rs much earlier, they still benefit from plenty of real-life experiences. They may be interested in the third R through counting games (counting buttons, stairs, trees... anything), rhymes like 'One, Two, Buckle my Shoe', and one-to-one matching activities (such as providing the right number of cups and saucers for five teddies at a tea party), but that doesn't mean it's necessary to move straight on to formal teaching.

There's plenty more physical, social, emotional and cognitive groundwork to be done if children are to be intrinsically motivated to learn rather than relying on adult direction. In terms of maths, a good kindergarten supports play-based learning by ensuring there are plenty of the best sort of 'concrete materials' available. Sandpits, piles of stones and gravel, bundles of sticks, paddling pools and water trays may not look like mathematical equipment, but the creative play they inspire is much more mathematically motivating than a worksheet full of sums. And trips to the woods, seaside and any other available wild places are more motivating still.

At present, there's interest among progressive UK and US educationists in something called Cognitively Guided Instruction, which mobilises the power of oral learning for five- and six-year-old children. The teacher provides a real-life problem (such as producing some tiny cakes and asking 'How can I share them out fairly between you?'), then invites the group to solve it. When the children come to a solution, they talk about the strategies each has used to get there. This discussion not only reveals where each child is in terms of mathematical understanding, helping the teacher see how best to support them in moving forward; it also gives children an opportunity to learn from each other, recognising which of their friends' strategies seem most effective. As a way of developing mathematical confidence and competence it seems to me eminently sensible ... but it takes time and the freedom for children to learn in this way – like infant scientists – through trial and error.

In fact, trial and error is what play is all about, and why it's such a powerful way of increasing children's potential as independent learners. The years between three and seven are very precious in this respect, as this is when children gradually develop their self-regulatory capacity. An education system can spend these years building on their natural motivation to explore the world and experiment with ways of thinking about mathematical concepts... or it can send them to school and provide ready-made formulae for getting ticks on a test paper.

Kindergarten practitioners can also develop children's mathematical understanding through specially designed lessons. Clare and David Mills, who made a Channel 4 documentary about European kindergarten practice, once gave me video footage of a Hungarian kindergarten teacher conducting a half-hour lesson with a group of six year olds. She kept them all thoroughly engaged with a mixture of songs, oral activities, games and two types of 'concrete' activity. The first involved building various constructions with large-scale three-dimensional shapes. The second was a series of number-representation tasks using little plastic rabbits, which were kept in bowls on the children's tables. The children each had a sheet of paper, on which to place the appropriate number of rabbits when the teacher gave a signal.

Since the VHS videotape was lost some years ago, I'm afraid the following description is based on memory, so can be taken with as many pinches of salt as you like, but it really impressed me at the time. First the teacher clapped eight times, so the children all fished out eight rabbits and lined them up. Then she blinked five times, so they lined up five rabbits. This seemed to me a great way of helping them internalise the 'feel' of numbers. Then she started on mental imagining tasks:

'Close your eyes and imagine you're under your table. Count how many legs it has. Put that many rabbits on the sheet.' The children fork out four rabbits. 'Now think how many legs there are for two tables. Imagine taking one of those legs away. How many are left? Put that many rabbits on your sheet.'

Children in Hungary don't do any written sums until they're seven, which is the same age as an English Year 2. A year after the video was made, David Mills asked the Hungarian class to sit the Year 2 maths SAT. Their scores far surpassed that year's average for England, where many children had been practising written sums since they were four. I suspect their lifelong confidence in the mental manipulation of numbers, shape, volume and so on will also outclass their English counterparts.

***

Recent changes in childhood experiences are influenced by a mathematical rule known as Moore's Law. Fifty years ago, Gordon Moore (one of the founders of Intel) predicted that the power and potential of digital technology would double roughly every two years. His 'law' has held true ever since, meaning that our culture has developed at an exponential rate. In a world moving at such electric speed, it's easy to forget that human development happens according to a biological timetable. The temptation to rush children through their childhood is immense – there's so much for them to learn these days that surely it's only sensible to get the three Rs under their belts as quickly as possible?

I hope this chapter has convinced you it isn't. Formal learning must still be built on age-old developmental foundations, and play is still children's inborn developmental learning drive. For most of the twentieth century, the early-start nations' attachment to premature schooling didn't cause too much damage because children were still playing in time-honoured ways at weekends, during school holidays and around the edges of every school day. But by the 1990s, 'real play' had begun to disappear and, combined with other fall-out from

Moore's Law, its loss has since left a growing number of children 'all over the place' in terms of conceptual development.

More and earlier schoolification is not a viable long-term answer to this socio-cultural phenomenon. Quite apart from the probable long-term consequences for the next generation's physical and mental health, there's now an ever-widening gap between children who manage to pass academic tests in spite of a high-pressure education system and those who fall by the wayside. The next chapter therefore considers the all-important social questions of why, despite eleven years of full-time education, around one third of British teenagers still fail to achieve a GCSE Grade C (the agreed mark of competence) in Maths and English... and why mental-health problems are mushrooming in teenagers of all abilities.

Chapter 5

MIND THE GAPS

Why early formal schooling widens the gap between rich and poor, how it also contributes to the gender gap and how a kindergarten approach could reduce inequality of every kind

If you want to do really well in the English educational system, there are three pieces of advice it would be sensible to follow:

- Choose well-educated parents with an income higher than the national average.
- Be female.
- Don't be born during the summer months.

This advice is based on long-standing statistics. Parental income and education have always conferred an educational advantage and – the world being as it is – probably always will. Girls have tended to outperform boys in the early stages of schooling since records began – and, in the past, marking systems in standardised tests were sometimes adjusted to even things up. And the youngest school entrants (in England, those who are just four when they start school in September) are less likely to be top of the class than older ones. These discrepancies have, sadly, become much more marked over the last twenty-five years.

The equality stakes

The problems of summerborns (and the youngest children in other early-start countries with different school entry dates) have received a fair bit of attention in recent years. There's now plenty of evidence that children who start school soon after their fourth birthday thrive less well throughout the education system than those who are nearing or over five at the beginning of the school year. This isn't surprising, as a year's difference when you're four years old amounts to a quarter of your entire time on earth. In 2015, in the face of fierce lobbying by the parents of summerborns, the English government instructed local authorities to allow them to defer school entry for their children. Since there are financial considerations involved, it remains to be seen how this relaxation of the rules works out or, due to the way deferment often operates, turns out to be damaging for children in other ways. And, of course, it only applies to summerborn children whose parents are prepared to go through the hoops of applying for deferment, which is usually the more-highly educated ones.

I've outlined the evidence about this issue in Appendix 5, partly because it's enmeshed in the detail of specific countries' entry dates, and partly because it distracts attention from *Upstart*'s central argument. Which is that all children – rich *and* poor, boys *and* girls, whatever their date of birth – would benefit from the raising of the school starting age and provision of three to four years of kindergarten education. This chapter deals with the equality stakes in terms of (1) family background and (2) gender.

Part One: Rich and Poor

Anyone living in the wealthy west can't fail to have noticed that wealth today is less evenly distributed than in the not-so-distant past. Indeed, according to a recent Oxfam report, five families now own more of the UK's wealth than the poorest 20 per cent of the entire population. The 'upwards social mobility', by which income was once distributed more fairly, ground to a halt thirty years ago and is now heading downwards. According to the Oxford sociologist who reported this trend, 'the emerging situation is one for which there is little historical precedent, and that carries potentially far-reaching political and wider social implications.' These wider social implications in 2015 included three and a half million children growing up in poverty in the UK, with another million estimated to join them by 2020.

Ethics and economics

Perhaps, like me, you find it morally repugnant that the sixth richest nation in the world should be sentencing so many of its children to lifelong disadvantage. Or maybe you simply recognise the economic argument that inequality is bad for everyone, rich and poor alike, and that one of the most effective ways to tackle it is national investment in the next generation. While I'd heartily agree with this economically inspired solution, I must point out that – even though this bit of the book is about wealth – 'investment in the next generation' doesn't mean the circumstances of disadvantaged children will be improved merely by throwing money at them.

During the first decade of the twenty-first century, a great deal of money was thrown at child poverty in the UK, with the intention of eliminating it by 2020. The New Labour government had accepted that 'early intervention' – between the ages of birth and three – is the key to breaking the cycle of disadvantage spawning a host of social evils, such as soaring demand for state benefits, increasing pressure on the NHS and a crisis in criminal justice that has British prisons bursting at the seams. The economic reason for targeting *child* poverty had been neatly summed up by Nobel prize-winner James Heckman: 'Every dollar invested in quality early childhood development for disadvantaged children produces a 7 per cent to 10 per cent return per year'.

While I'm all for supporting disadvantaged families as much as humanly possible, I wished right from the start that this supposedly humanitarian crusade wasn't based on the slogan 'It's the economy, stupid.' Little children are not mere elements in a fiscal equation – they're living, breathing human beings – but as long as politicians are locked in a purely economic mindset their concept of 'quality early child development' won't take account of four-letter words like 'love' and 'play'. In fact, I'm convinced there's a fundamental flaw in the financial equation that's underpinned these 'interventions' from the start. With one hand, the government was welcoming tax revenues from companies whose products damage children's mental and physical health; with the other, they put this money into projects designed to improve children's mental and physical health. If politicians are really serious about improving disadvantaged children's lives, why not start by regulating the markets in junk food, junk play and 'Yuk and Wow' screen-based entertainment for tots?

It also worries me that interventions driven by purely economic arguments are inevitably blighted by the need for endless measurement and accountability procedures, to check they're giving 'value for money'. As I travel around the country on the childhood research trail, I meet professionals in a wide variety of children's services and, especially in disadvantaged areas, they are universally exhausted by mushrooming workloads combined with mountains of bureaucracy. This leaves them with neither time nor energy to engage satisfactorily with the families they're trying to help. There's no way that tackling the fallout of 'toxic childhood syndrome' can be micro-managed by politicians and civil servants sitting comfortably in government offices.

There's also, of course, the problem of the cost. The most successful initiatives introduced by New Labour, such as the Family Nurse Partnership,[10] tend to be expensive in terms of personnel so

---

10 A highly personalised intervention, in which specially trained health visitors support disadvantaged families before, and for a year or so after, a new baby's birth, modelling successful parent–child interaction. I've heard it described as 'mothering the mothers'.

can't be widely introduced. This sort of effective intervention has therefore proved a mere drop in the ocean of social and cultural disadvantage. Also, as economist Leon Feinstein has pointed out, the positive effects of support in the earliest stages of children's lives soon disappear unless the support is continued. In England, twenty-first-century political 'support' for children of three and over has so far resulted in increasing schoolification of early years education. So I'm not at all surprised that public investment in early intervention hasn't paid off and millions of pounds of tax-payers' money have been effectively wasted (not to mention all the blood, sweat and tears of various caring professionals).

A global financial crisis in 2008, followed by a change of government in 2010, led to dwindling availability of public funds, and current attempts to stem the tide of disadvantage in England's children rely largely on private investment. However, New Labour's decade-long exercise in state-sponsored money-shovelling clearly illustrated that genuine social change requires an ethical as well as an economic investment – politicians must value the human strengths required to help disadvantaged children, not just the money that pays for them. Professor Richard Layard of the London School of Economics is one of many leading academics who've embraced this argument, and his department now stresses the importance of human wellbeing in a nation's economic success. He summed up the change of mindset required in an interview for *Toxic Childhood*: 'We have to change the relative prestige accorded to smart-arsed behaviour and that accorded to kindness.'

The smart-arsed slogan 'It's the economy, stupid' is a highly inadequate basis for a nation's political life. While the economy is clearly important for everyone's material wellbeing, ethical values matter too. There are some things that money just can't buy, and the key ingredients of healthy early child development – love and play – are two of them. So let's forget about smart-arsed initiatives for a moment and try a little kindly intended, highly personal, human attunement.

A tale of under-achievement?

Imagine you're a 'severely disadvantaged child', just setting off for nursery school. Since your parents are extremely strapped for cash, your life has been riven with difficulties since the moment you were born. You've probably spent your earliest years in a cramped, dilapidated home in a run-down inner-city area with few local shops or other amenities. Maybe it was damp, poorly heated, with inadequate cooking, living and/or sleeping facilities. It certainly didn't have a back garden to play in and the nearest play park is usually covered in broken glass, dog poo and discarded hypodermic needles, so your mum gives it a wide berth.

Due to the ongoing cycle of poverty, your parents were probably raised in similar circumstances, so there's a good chance they by now suffer from a variety of physical and/or mental health problems which, like their neighbours, they may be 'self-medicating' with alcohol or drugs. This combination of poverty and substance abuse means the rates of violence and criminal activity in your neighbourhood are high, so you find out very early how scary the world can be. You may even be witnessing violence in your own home.

Your mum is more likely than most mums to be depressed. She may also be constantly exhausted from working long hours in a low-paid, insecure job (or from trying to scrape by on benefits) and she's certainly beset by the multiple problems of raising a child in poverty. This doesn't mean she loves you any less than other mothers love their little ones, but it does mean that your first three years on earth were very unlike those described in 'Birth–three' in Chapter 2. In the worst-case scenario, mum might not have managed to keep you adequately fed, clothed, warm and safe. Even if she succeeded in rising to these daily challenges, she was unlikely to have much time or energy left for the emotional input babies and toddlers need.

So instead of tuning into your inborn need for interaction with real people and the real world, your mum probably tuned you into an electronic babysitter for much of the day, while herself escaping into the much more congenial world of daytime TV or Facebook chat. Like the babies in Sally Ward's research, you didn't learn how to listen to the human voice during your earliest months and, like the disdvantaged toddlers studied by American researchers Betty Hart and Todd Risley, you were exposed during your pre-school years to around 80 per cent less real-life spoken language than 'lucky' children. Your mum was, though, desperate to keep you as safe as possible so you've probably spent most of your life so far strapped into baby seats of some kind and seldom had the chance to move around freely. Since it wasn't safe to play outdoors either, you missed out almost entirely on opportunities for active, exploratory, self-initiated play.

Consequently, you've arrived at nursery school today with attention and language skills that are way below the average level. Your conceptual understanding and problem-solving ability are also extremely low level, your physical development is poor and your social skills are negligible. (How could they be anything else, when none of the adults or children you've met so far have modelled the sort of social skills required in a nursery?) Emotionally, you're pretty fragile. While your family probably moved heaven and earth to provide some consumerist love tokens (techno-toys, fashion clothing, Disney tie-ins and so on), they've also passed on deep feelings of inadequacy driven by their own lack of social status. This means that, when they talk to you, their words are twice as likely to be discouraging as encouraging. It's not that they *want* to lower your self-esteem, just that for most of their lives they've heard little but discouragement themselves. Unconsciously, unintentionally, they're passing on an emotional inheritance of low self-confidence and lack of hope for the future.

It's a sorry tale and it's been going on remorselessly for generations. But it doesn't have to have an unhappy ending. The good news is that, despite this catalogue of early misadventure, *you're* not beaten yet. It takes a great deal of misery and failure to destroy the human spirit, especially a fresh young human spirit like yours, bursting with the potential to learn. At three years old, you're still capable of responding positively to kindness and support from adults at the nursery and thus acquiring those much-vaunted social, linguistic and attention skills.

You're also still keen to explore and experiment, which means you can discover the delights of physical activity, emotional engagement and creative play. Given your lack of social awareness, the activities that delight and engage you in the early stages of pre-school education may not be very acceptable but – with plenty of sensitive support from understanding adults – you'll gradually suss out the difference between constructive play and destructive mischief. And, as you get used to socialising with other children, you'll also discover that it's well worth sticking by mutually agreed rules.

Of course, given the experiences of your first three years, it'll take at least another three to unlearn old habits of behaviour and pick up all these demanding new skills, concepts and manners. But, with sensitive care from highly attuned nursery practitioners and plenty of opportunities for real play (particularly outdoors) you could – by the age of about seven – have developed the powers of self-regulation required to take full advantage of your school career. History has shown that even children with innumerable early social handicaps *can* develop the personal confidence to become successful learners, break out of the poverty cycle, grow up into responsible citizens and make a valuable contribution to the society that supported them. A tale of early under-achievement *can* end happily ever after.

This is not to suggest that governments should stop investing in effective early years interventions, nor that a developmentally appropriate kindergarten system is the answer to all the problems a small disadvantaged child will encounter as time goes on. A civilised country should also be committed to improving the living conditions of disadvantaged families in any way it can. But, in the twenty-first century, an effective system of early childcare and education is probably the single most effective way of breaking the cycle of disadvantage by providing a level educational playing field for *all* its children.

A tale of dwindling achievement

Sadly, the good news is yet to happen, because in early-start countries support for all-round development – which is what disadvantaged children need most of all – now takes second place to 'readiness' for phonics and sums from the day they turn four. The government has naturally assembled a mountain of data to prove their policy works, and politicians take great pride in the short-term academic gains to be gleaned from the structured learning programmes they introduce (for example, see section 'Huckt on Fonix' in Chapter 4). However, as far as I can discover, there is no evidence – from anywhere, at any time – to suggest these short-term gains are anything but temporary.

During the 1960s and 70s, there were many attempts to improve the educational achievement of disadvantaged pre-schoolers in the USA, but very few achieved significant long-term gains. One of the most successful was the Abecedarian Project in North Carolina, which started from birth and incorporated parent education, health, and nutrition as well as early learning programmes starting when children were four or five. The programmes involved educational games, tailored to children's individual developmental needs, which focused on social, emotional and cognitive development, with particular emphasis on language. In fact, the 'early intervention' component of the Abecedarian Project sounds like an early version of the Family Nurse Partnership and the pre-school activities sound very like the sort of short teacher-led sessions that are normal in European kindergartens

Other projects concentrated on formal instruction for pre-schoolers. The most successful of these – a system of oral drill called Direct Instruction – appeared to enhance children's progress until, in the words of one of its fans, 'at minimum second grade'. Unfortunately, no one followed those children's progress through beyond the age of eight so we'll never know whether that fan was right to add 'and likely longer.' However, the few longitudinal studies available suggest that, for disadvantaged children, early academic gains disappear by the time the children reach secondary school.

For instance, in a 2002 US study comparing children from poor families who attended 'academic' pre-schools with others from the same background who attended 'child-initiated' pre-schools, the academic teaching paid off in the first couple of years, but there was a dramatic reversal of fortunes as time went on. By the age of ten, the difference in educational achievement between the two groups had evened out and a year later, children whose pre-school experiences had been academically directed earned significantly lower grades than children who had attended child-initiated pre-school classes.

This knits up with evidence now emerging from from the *Harvard Centre for the Developing Child* about the role of those age-old ingredients, love and play, in the nurture of resilience during the early years. 'Resilience' is the term used by psychologists to describe an individual's ability to weather stressful experiences and 'bounce back' from difficulties.

Although 'top-down' teaching in the early years gives children an academic head start, it also affects their long-term emotional resilience. As time goes on, their greater susceptibility to stress can lead to poorer, rather than increased achievement. In today's high-pressure educational culture, youngsters need all the resilience they can muster, and children whose home circumstances add further sources of stress would especially benefit from as many resilience-nurturing experiences as possible during the kindergarten years. While lack of emotional resilience is probably not the only reason why early academic gains 'wash out' by children's teens, a longitudinal report published in 2015 indicated that support during the early years for social and emotional development is a signficant protective factor.

Misreading the evidence

This conclusion is supported by a longitudinal study of American children from disadvantaged backgrounds that started in the late 1960s. The High/Scope Perry Project followed the educational progress of three groups of five year olds randomly allocated to different types of pre-school provision:

1. direct instruction
2. informal free play activities
3. a combination of free play and short structured sessions of teacher-mediated talk (a High/Scope kindergarten approach).

As you'd expect, Group (1) started school at an academic advantage. But during their subsequent school careers nearly half of them needed special help for social behaviour issues, compared with only six per cent in the other two groups. While the academic achievement of all three groups was similar, children from Group (1) were twice as likely to be expelled as those from the other two groups. By the time they were 23 years old, police records showed that 34 per cent of this first group had been arrested for felony, compared with nine per cent of the others.

In a TV interview in the late 1990s, chief High/Scope researcher David Weikhart reported that, during their twenties, Group (1) children were also involved in more disruption in the community because 'they found people like shopkeepers, landlords and clerks in stores gave them a hard time.' He explained that they also reported poorer relationships with their families, were less likely to be married and had more difficulty holding down jobs than members of Groups (2) and (3). Since all the children in the High/Scope project had the same type of home background, it appears that play-based, developmentally appropriate pre-school experiences had long-term effects in terms of social adjustment and emotional resilience.

I was therefore astonished, during a radio broadcast a couple of years ago, when a fellow-participant claimed long-standing US research had proved that 'structured teaching' is better than play for disadvantaged children's long-term social development, and even more astonished when he cited the High/Scope Perry Project. Our discussion deteriorated into a spirited 'Oh yes it does – Oh no it doesn't' exchange, which wasn't much help to the listeners. Afterwards, I went back to check out the High/Scope study and try to work out how he might have misinterpreted it.

Write-ups of the High/Scope experiment gloss over the fact that Group (2) children – who went to a 'free-play' nursery – did as well in the social and emotional stakes as those who attended a High/Scope kindergarten (which isn't surprising, as the authors had their own system to promote). I suspect my radio opponent, who wasn't an educationist, was misled by words like 'structured' and 'teacher' in the description of High/Scope methodology, so leapt to the conclusion that it involved 'structured teaching'. In fact, High/Scope pre-schools are essentially play-based and their short sessions of teacher-mediated talk ('Plan-Do-Review') are similar to the sort of animated conversations between children and practitioners you'd see in any good kindergarten, anywhere in the world.

I can only suppose that the politicians behind the current schoolification of early childhood in England labour under similar misconceptions about what 'quality early education' looks like. If formal instruction worked, the schoolifed approach to early years that's been *in situ* in the UK for well over a decade should by now be delivering noticeable improvement in our teenagers' exam results. Sadly, the 'long tail of under-achievement' (the 33% of children who fail to get a C in GCSE Maths and English) is still with us and is still disproportionately composed of children from economically deprived backgrounds.

So far, this has resulted in the application of firmer and fiercer pressure on primary schools to focus on tests and targets, along with political denunciation of secondary schools for failing to maintain children's 'progress'. Strangely, no matter how much governments tinker with the system, nothing seems to improve the situation.

Smart-arsed, selfish and smug

So here's a smart-arsed suggestion for closing the attainment gap in early-start nations. How about introducing well-resourced Finnish-type kindergartens for under-privileged children up to the age of seven, while leaving the privileged kids to carry on putting their noses to the grindstone at four or five? With time and support to catch up on all-round development, including communication skills, the disadvantaged children would have a much greater chance of doing well at school, and also be better fitted to put their education to good use once they reach the workplace. Over the years, that should help even things up a bit in terms of income distribution.

It would not, however, be either ethical or kind. In a world where play is being squeezed out of all children's lives, enlightened adults should be doing everything possible to ensure that every child enjoys an unhurried childhood. And in the long run, society is more likely to prosper if *all* children's early educational experiences involve opportunities for healthy physical and mental development. For instance, if more time were available to support the social and emotional development of children from wealthier homes, they might find it easier in adulthood to empathise with the plight of the poor – and they might even, like the citizens of Nordic countries, be prepared to pay more in taxes to create a fairer state.

Sadly at present, a notable decline in empathy has been spotted among American college students (youngsters who, thanks to the achievement gap, are more likely to hail from privileged than under-privileged backgrounds). Many of their *almae matres* require them to complete 'attitude' questionnaires. On items such as 'I often have tender, concerned feelings for people less fortunate than me' and 'I try to look at everybody's side in a disagreement before I make a decision', students in 2010 were almost 75 per cent less likely to answer 'Yes' than those in 1980. Psychology professor Jean Twenge points out that today's college students are also more self-satisfied and narcissistic than their predecessors – they're 30 per cent more likely to tick questionnaire responses such as 'I always know what I am doing' and 'I like to be the centre of attention' than their counterparts forty years ago.

There could be lots of explanations for these changing attitudes: increasing social isolation due to screen-based lifestyles; the culture of self-promotion normalised by social networking; a market-induced obsession with body image and appearance; changes in parenting strategies, and so on. All are likely to be significant factors but, given the knock-on effects of early childhood experiences on long-term human development, the USA's increasingly early start on formal education must surely be implicated. The foundations of any adult's sense of identity – including his or her social attitudes and self-image – are laid during the first seven years, so children for whom cognitive achievement is emphasised at the expense of social and emotional development are more likely to be particularly vulnerable to other damaging factors in an increasingly selfish, materialistic culture.

I've so far found no statistical evidence of similar attitudinal changes in other early-start nations but there seems no reason to believe that privileged young people across our global consumerist culture are very different from those in the States. There are certainly regular complaints from UK employers that many graduate recruits display an inflated sense of entitlement and have difficulties working within a team. They also complain about young employees' lack of determination, patience, and ability to think outside the box ('He's got a first class degree from a top university,' a CEO recently told me, 'but when a problem cropped up the other day, d'you know what he did? He phoned his mum!'). All the aforesaid qualities, incidentally, are nurtured during children's early years through opportunities for play.

Poor little rich kids

Throughout *Upstart*, I've stressed that developmentally appropriate kindergarten education isn't merely a preparation for formal schooling but for life. And, since all the parents I meet (rich and poor) claim they want their children to live happy lives, it's worth noting that a recent report on wellbeing from the London School of Economics concluded that 'the key to future happiness' is emotional health in childhood.

There's no doubt that a certain level of material prosperity can help maintain a child's emotional health, but it's by no means the only ingredient. Children from well-heeled families are just as vulnerable to the effects of emotional neglect as those from the other side of the tracks and if, as a teacher in a very expensive preparatory school once put it, 'mummy and daddy are both out earning shed-loads of money, and the kids are looked after by an au pair... who just takes them to special classes or sticks them in their bedrooms with the telly and the computer' it's bound to affect their emotional development. Wealthy parents these days are often unaware of the importance of love, time and attention for young children (perhaps because they didn't experience much of it themselves). Just like their disadvantaged counterparts, they are often in thrall to the message that love is mainly a matter of spending money. But as well as buying their offspring technological toys, designer clothing and so on, wealthy parents can also invest heavily in education. These days this means pushing their children to achieve at an ever earlier age.

The Managing Director of a London educational consultancy recently explained that, 'if the goal for your child is Oxford, Cambridge or a Russell Group university, it's about tracing that back to the very start and considering what the best route might be.' This has intensified the competition for places in prestigious nursery schools – the ones with a good record of getting children into prestigious preparatory schools, which in turn may help them into prestigious independent secondary schools, from which there's much better chance of proceeding to a prestigious university. Nowadays, there are waiting lists for 'elite' nursery schools in the UK and USA, wealthy parents are advised to enrol their children into the best pre-preps while they're still *in utero*, and tutoring services are available for two and three year olds.

Over the last fifteen years, many teachers in independent prep and pre-prep schools have told me of their concern about the long-term effects on pupils' wellbeing of pressure from home for academic achievement. As the parental anxiety kicks in earlier and earlier, the effects of this pressure may not be as immediately obvious as in the six-year-old boy described by an independent school headmistress ('clinically depressed: crying, withdrawn, and waking early, tearful... very bright but so anxious he was blocked'), but it will inevitably affect overall development, including long-term resilience. Excessive stress in any child's formative years impacts on emotional health and (as mentioned in the section 'More haste, more problems' in Chapter 1) the most recent long-term study to link early formal schooling with lifelong mental health issues didn't focus on disadvantaged children but on middle-class Californians who were 'intelligent and good learners'.

The ethos of a market-driven, winners-and-losers educational system is completely at odds with what we know **all** children need in their earliest years. So I believe there are profound social implications in the constant ratcheting up of competitive pressure for 'advantaged children':

- As the hot-housing virus increasingly infects wealthy parents, their behaviour has knock-on effects on 'aspirational' parents across all social classes, as well as on politicians who are already committed to early schoolification.
- The children of 'aspirational' parents of all social classes are likely to be the leaders and opinion formers of the future. If the definition of 'aspiration' involves neglecting emotional health and social responsibility in the pursuit of ever-earlier academic achievement, we can wave goodbye to the possibility of ever achieving social justice.

***

Young children, whatever their economic circumstances, are entirely at the mercy of their parents. As far as they're concerned, the way mum and dad demonstrate their love is what 'love' means – even when it involves being left for hours with a computer game or booked in for incomprehensible tutoring sessions. If adults don't support the under-sevens in playing the way nature intended them to play, they've no alternative but to turn their back on nature and comply with whatever the grown-ups expect.

Given the influence of global corporations on national governments, I don't imagine politicians will dare do much to rein in the pernicious influence of market forces on the way parents demonstrate love to their children. But they could do something to influence the way children play and the quality of out-of-home care and education in the pre-school years. Raising the school starting age and providing a developmentally appropriate play-based kindergarten stage could:

- support the all-round development of all children in the state sector
- provide every state-educated child, no matter what his or her background, with the best possible start to formal education.

And since that should increase the sum of human happiness *and* contribute to social justice, it seems to me a no-brainer.

Incidentally, in 2015, the Nordic countries – Sweden, Finland, Norway, Denmark and Iceland – are the most economically egalitarian nations on earth and all regularly appear in the top ten of the United Nations annual World Happiness Report (the UK currently languishes in twenty-first place). Coincidentally, the Nordic nations all have long-established, well-resourced kindergarten systems.

Part Two: Boys and Girls

Ever since I started banging on about raising the school starting age, the people who've shown the most interest are the parents of three- to seven-year-old boys. Many small boys tend, for reasons to be explained in the rest of this chapter, to find school life distinctly uncongenial. As one mum recently put it: within a few weeks of her son starting in the reception class, 'The light went out in his eyes.'

It must be admitted that male aversion to formal education is nothing new. There's a description of a disaffected schoolboy on a Sumerian tablet, Shakespeare's archetypal boy-child crept 'unwillingly to school' and Wordsworth described how, once schooling begins, 'shades of the prison house begin to close around the growing boy'.

The educational gender gap is a global phenomenon, and the problem of boys' achievement (at least in literacy) is an issue in later-start as well as early-start countries, though the former seem to be dealing with it rather more successfully than the latter. After a century or so of female access to education, it's clear that girls are far more likely to flourish at school than boys. However, the female advantage soon disappears once they enter the male-dominated world of work – at which point the gender gap in achievement is suddenly reversed. So could something about both sexes' early experiences of learning be involved?

Nature, nuture and gender

'Girls have been faster learners for six million years!' proclaimed a newspaper headline, sending me scurrying to the journal *Nature*, to check out research about chimpanzees passing on cultural knowledge to their young. Apparently, adult chimps show their offspring how to harvest termites, which are a useful source of protein if there's nothing better to eat. The mother chimp (for it is she who nurtures the little ones) selects a strong reed, inserts it into a termite mound, wiggles it around a bit, then carefully pulls it out... to reveal a termite lolly.

Little girl chimps watch this procedure with rapt concentration, and are soon selecting reeds for themselves and trying to copy the routine. Little boy chimps tend to watch for a while, then lose interest and run off to play-fight, play-hunt and scramble about in the trees. This is, of course, as one would expect according to their pre-determined gender roles: the males are preparing through their play to be hunters; the females (who'll spend their adult lives either pregnant or carrying a baby chimp) are less interested in active, exploratory activities and more inclined to imitate their grown-up carers.

Our species' cultural evolution means that very few human males now spend their lives hunting and few females in western countries are primarily engaged in child-rearing. We've therefore devised educational systems to provide equal opportunities for both sexes. But, since play is children's natural learning mechanism, they're learning from play long before they start formal education, and anyone who's watched small children play knows that the behaviour of human infants is startlingly similar to that of the chimpanzees in the study.

So why do little boys tend to be distractable, rumbustious and exploratory in their play, while little girls are much more likely to behave in ways that mimic their (generally female) adult carers? Do the very young of both sexes play differently because

- there are deep-seated biological differences between the way male and female humans think and act, related to their respective roles in reproduction, which are unlikely to go away just because the culture changes?
- adults are influenced by long-established gender stereotypes that they unconsciously pass on to children so that, despite our cultural evolution, stereotypical behaviour still lingers on?

And what are the implications for early years education?

As someone who trained as a teacher in the 1970s, I arrived in the classroom convinced that 'gender is a cultural concept'. Like many adults of the time, I was often deeply frustrated by children's irritating tendency to abide by stereotypes – despite our bans on toy weapons, small boys ingeniously turned anything that came to hand into 'pretend' swords and guns, and although we provided carefully selected, gender-neutral toys, small girls tended to wrap them up in blankets and cradle them like dolls. We were similarly appalled by less-well-informed adults' insistence on treating the two sexes differently from the moment they were born, praising boys for being 'big' and 'strong' and girls for being 'sweet' and 'pretty'.

However, by the 1990s it did seem that, despite these early introductions to gender stereotyping, the sexual equality project in western democracies was well on track. Girls were flourishing in the educational system and expected to be economically independent adults on equal footing with men. Since laws had been established to ensure equal opportunities in the workplace, it seemed we could stop worrying about children's play, concentrate on stamping out the remaining vestiges of adult sexism and all would be well. Twenty years later, however, things aren't looking so hopeful. Although most women are at work, they earn less than men and have far fewer of the top jobs; they're also more likely than their male counterparts to be taking on the unpaid work of home-making and child-rearing. At the same time, many boys are failing to reach their educational potential, which makes a significant contribution to the widening achievement gap in early-start countries and leaves many young men under-educated, out of work and often extremely angry.

The more I discover about early child development, the more I'm convinced that society's failure in all these respects is due to our lack of respect for biology. There are sound developmental reasons why young male chimps behave as they do in the *Nature* article, and why little boys take to early schooling less willingly than little girls. They stem from the well-established fact that, in general, the male of the species lags behind the female in developmental terms from birth, a difference that doesn't really even out until early adulthood. So little boys – on the whole – are more likely to be distractible than little girls and take longer to socialise.

If carers and teachers cater for this general developmental delay, it shouldn't affect either sex's potential for success at school, nor for participating on entirely equal terms in society during adulthood. On the other hand, if we ignore it, the long-term effects (coupled with other twenty-first-century cultural phenomena) are likely to perpetuate old-fashioned gender-stereotyping and seriously undermine the quest for sexual equality.

My personal interest in gender and child development was inspired by that article in *Nature*. Apparently, the little-boy chimps' distractibility doesn't worry the adult chimps at all. They just carry on taking the kids down to the termite mounds and showing them how to harvest termites. Eventually, the small male hunters drift back from their active play long enough to learn the skills of termite-lolly manufacture, just like their sisters. But apparently it takes them roughly twice as long as the girl chimps to acquire the relevant small-scale motor skills and they interrupt what they're doing four times as often.

When I tell early years practitioners about this research, their reaction is one of wry amusement, mixed with sadness. They recognise the statistics and would love the luxury of time and space for their small, male, primate learners to develop the self-regulatory skills required for the three Rs as willingly as their as female classmates.

The trouble with gender

Apart from the developmental delay, science tells us that a child's sex shouldn't be an issue during childhood. While sex hormones are necessarily active *in utero* in order to determine whether the baby is male or female, they go into hibernation shortly after the birth and thereafter exercise minimal influence on children's lives until they reach puberty. As developmental psychologist Elizabeth Spelke points out, in their first year of life, boys and girls in scientific studies don't demonstrate particularly 'gendered' interests: 'Infants don't divide up the labour of understanding the world with males focusing on mechanics and females on emotions. Male and female infants are interested in both objects and people, and learn about both.'

Other scientists claim there's as much variation in terms of 'gendered' behaviour across the members of one sex as there is between boys and girls on the whole. To put that in stereotypical terms, some little girls behave more 'boyishly' than others (they're noisier, more active and/or less interested in other people's emotions) while some little boys have characteristics that are considered more 'girlish' (quieter, more contained in their play and/or more sensitive to people's feelings) and these variations are greater than the difference between the 'average boy' and the 'average girl'.

The current consensus among psychologists seems to be that, although children are fully aware of their own sex by the time they're two, the concept of gender as a permanent characteristic (something that can't be changed by making superficial adjustments to appearance) isn't fully formed until they're six or seven. This means that, even though children are surrounded by gender stereotypes from birth, during the kindergarten years it *should* be possible for them to learn that traditionally 'girlish' or 'boyish' behaviour isn't the province of one or other sex – just part of everyone's potential human repertoire. Of course, being children, the main way they'll internalise these messages is through the power of play.

However, there are two significant twenty-first-century cultural developments that make it difficult for children to accept non-gendered variations in personality. First, in a screen-saturated culture, they're constantly exposed to commercially driven gender stereotypes from a very early age (the 'pretty princess' stereotype for girls versus the 'naughty superhero' stereotype for boys). This inevitably affects their understanding of how males and females are expected to behave. Secondly, attempts to establish sexual equality in the workplace have taken little account of the impact on family life of having two parents in paid work, so young children from 'hard-working families' can miss out on real-life care and attention during the years when love and play are hugely important for their sense of identity. In this case, they may well be overly influenced by the images of stereotypical femininity and masculinity portrayed in the media.

Yet if equality is to be achieved, society must prepare both boys and girls to rise above the stereotypes, and support both sexes in developing *all* the human strengths they'll need in a (hopefully) increasingly equal society. That means nurturing the empathy both boys and girls will require in the future for successful child-rearing themselves, as well as the resilience and can-do attitude required for success in the workplace. In this, there's clearly an important role for kindergarten practitioners who influence children's social and emotional development at a formative stage in their lives. In the rest of this chapter, I'll outline some of the main gender issues currently plaguing education in the UK, and their connection to what happens in children's earliest years.

The trouble with boys ...

The 'boy problem' has been high on the educational agenda for several decades. In England, where all five year olds had their progress recorded on the Foundation Stage Profile between 2000 and 2015, girls out-performed boys in every category from 2008 onwards. They then maintained their lead throughout the educational system and now have more chance than boys, first of getting to university, then of graduating at the end of the course. Around 50 per cent of women are now expected to have a degree by the age of 30, but only 40 per cent of men.

So what's behind this educational descent of man? Well, for one thing, all the developmental disorders listed in the section called 'The special needs expolosion' in Chapter 3 are more prevalent in boys than girls: dyslexia is around three times more common, ADHD and dyspraxia four times, and boys are *nine* times more likely to be diagnosed with ASD. So as these conditions have increased, more boys are educationally disadvantaged.

The male of the species is generally more 'fragile' than the female from the word 'Go', with a greater likelihood of miscarriage, premature birth and developmental disorders. This seems to be related to the activation of the Y chromosome at around eight weeks after conception, which also causes the slight developmental delay. Once babies are born, this small developmental gap between the sexes widens, at least in terms of social maturation, and is clearly evident by age three or four (see also 'The power to please', below). If, as outlined in Chapter 3, modern lifestyles exacerbate developmental delay, the average boy probably needs more 'mothering' than the average girl to compensate. Similarly, there's good reason for providing boys with the type of highly attuned nurture available in a developmentally appropriate kindergarten before requiring them to knuckle down to schoolwork. They'll particularly benefit from plenty of opportunities for social play, to support language and interpersonal skills.

It's widely agreed that problems with boys' educational achievement are connected with issues around masculinity in a rapidly changing, consumer-driven world. While many of the old stereotypes of 'manliness' no longer apply in a supposedly sexually equal society, they're still fiercely promoted through commercial channels. Marketers target young male consumers through the 'cool' attractions of power, domination and risk-taking, starting with Spiderman costumes and gradually pointing them towards action films and (often violent) computer games. Accordingly, a damaging male counter-culture often develops in schools and is nowadays even noticeable – in embryonic form – at pre-school level.

When consumer culture drives a gender divide from the moment children are born, boys soon learn to define themselves as *not-girls* and vice versa. Membership of the male peer group then depends not only on being tough and edgy, but also on being *not-girl* – and now that girls are doing so well in the educational stakes, academic success is increasingly associated with *girliness*. Unless schools are able to counter this tendency, it means that the better girls perform in class or exams, the less value is attached to school achievement by the male 'peer police'. As time goes on, even academically able boys can be adversely affected when they have to choose between fitting in with the other lads or being labelled 'girly' or 'gay'.

The schoolification of early childhood seriously exacerbates the male–female educational divide. Since boys lag behind girls developmentally, it's not surprising that five-year-old boys also lag behind girls in terms of scores on the Foundation Profile. Asking small boys to perform tasks that are developmentally beyond them is setting them up to fail, and failure at such an impressionable age is likely to have an impact on the male psyche, not least in terms of attitude to school.[11]

By giving them a couple more years in which to mature – socially, emotionally and cognitively – we could ensure that all boys have the best possible chance to fulfil their academic potential, which might help the male 'peer police' amend their attitude to education.

Not surprisingly, the confusion about the meaning of masculinity has coincided with growing concerns about mental health among young males. In 2006, the British Medical Association reported that boys in the five- to ten-year-old age group were twice as likely as girls to have an emotional, behavioural or mental health problem, while in the ten- to fifteen-year-old age group 11 per cent of boys had diagnosable conditions as opposed to 8 per cent of girls.

---

11 We shouldn't kid ourselves that small children aren't aware of things like national test results. I've heard six year olds singing about it in the playground: 'Girls go to college to get more knowledge; boys go to Jupiter to get more stupider.'

... and the trouble with girls

However, when I questioned educational psychologists about this trend in mental health statistics they tended to be sceptical. Dr Sammi Timimi, a specialist in boys' development, summed up their reasons: 'The big difference is that boys externalise their problems and it comes out as bad behaviour – girls tend to internalise them, as sadness.' Perhaps, they suggested, it was just taking longer for people to notice the results of the gender identity crisis in young women than in young men.

Sure enough, more recent statistics show that emotional and mental health problems have become at least as common among female teenagers as male ones. The consumer-driven emphasis on fashion and appearance for girls at a very young age means that body-image problems now start as early as five or six. The steady sexualisation of society and the increasingly violent and misogynistic nature of internet porn also have an effect on girls' self-image and behaviour. And many academically able girls are also finding it difficult to cope with the constant pressure to excel in tests and exams, which seems to start earlier with every passing year. In 2015, research suggested that a tenth of fifteen year olds (mostly female) were suffering from an eating disorder, while a fifth were self-harming. These figures are also increasing year on year.

In the section above titled 'A tale of dwindling achievement', I explained how mental health issues are often linked to a lack of resilience, which psychologists believe can be strength-ened during children's early life by the usual developmental combination of parental love and real play, particularly active outdoor play. I'd therefore like to see more attention paid to the possible connection between girls' early success in formal learning and their declining interest in physical activity and sport as childhood progresses. Perhaps, while celebrating girls' early academic progress, we've ignored the fact that it comes at the expense of active outdoor play. This lack of play may, in the long run, have significant reprecussions in terms of health and wellbeing.

I suspect the question of acquired resilience (and other personal characteristics developed through active, exploratory play) could help account for another gender-based phenomenon. It's increasingly apparent that, however well girls do at school, once they hit the workplace equality is still largely beyond their grasp. In 2010, there was a fresh outburst of feminist literature with titles like *Living Dolls: The return of sexism* and *The Equality Illusion*. While these suggested many reasons why the sexual-equality project has run into stormy waters, they gave little consideration to the potential ill-effects of children's early experiences of gender-stereotyping.

Indeed, if I hadn't been immersed for so long in the literature on child development, I probably wouldn't have dreamed of connecting teenagers' problems with their early childhood experiences, let alone pondering whether an early school starting age might be involved in continued female inequality at work and women's failure to make any noticeable impression on the famous glass ceiling. If something is a grown-up problem, it's obvious to hunt for 'grown-up' explanations, usually economic or political ones. But while politics and economics are undoubtedly important factors, the psychological mindset of a nation depends on the way its children are reared.

Gender is fundamental to self-image, so gender-specific differences in children's attitudes to learning are bound to have long-term effects. If an early-start policy puts many boys off schoolwork before they've really begun, it will inevitably affect attitudes to masculinity, making young males increasingly vulnerable to commercialised 'bad boy' stereotypes. And if, despite girls' early success at school, their early education doesn't equip them to thrive in the world of work or in their social and personal lives outside school, then we need to look with a highly questioning eye at what all this early pressure for desk-bound learning actually achieves. It isn't leading to workplace success. If it were, girls would dominate the workplace. And it doesn't seem to be leading to resilience or happiness either.

The power to please

There is, according to neuroscientists, no evidence that females are cleverer than males or vice versa. Even scientists who favour the influence of nature over nurture accept this. Some evolutionary biologists (largely a male breed) argue that there are more males in the 'genius' category of certain scientific subjects, but acknowledge that this is balanced by the presence of more males at the opposite end of the intellectual scale. ('More prodigies, more idiots', as one cheerfully put it.) However, there's one small nugget of information about very early development that could be highly significant in terms of girls' early school achievement – and unusually, there seems to be no dispute about it, even between male evolutionary biologists and female developmental psychologists. It's a very tiny gender difference to start with, but it sets off a chain reaction that – unless we find ways to address it – could perpetuate unhelpful gender stereotypes forever.

On the day they're born, all babies (male and female) try to focus on adult human faces – not surprisingly, since they rely on those adults to keep them alive. However, over the next three months, girl babies on average become about four times better than boys at focusing their gaze in this way. This gives them a very small early advantage in terms of encouraging adults to gaze back, thus establishing the dance of communication that underpins early attachment and attunement (see Chapter 2).

This probably explains why girls are generally quicker than boys to imitate various sorts of social behaviour – as they and their carers keep rewarding each other, they get more practice in imitation. On average, baby girls copy facial expressions (such as raising their eyebrows and widening their eyes to greet an approaching adult) slightly earlier than boys, then gestures such as raising their arms to be picked up and waving bye-bye. As time goes on, they also start talking sooner and increase their vocabulary more quickly. There are, of course, many advantages to early social awareness, especially in an early-start country, so it's not surprising that girls settle into school faster or that, by the age of four, most are ready and willing to imitate adults when they demonstrate specific literacy and numeracy skills. But there's also a significant disadvantage – a sociable child is more likely than an unsociable one to become a lifelong people-pleaser.

The ability to balance other people's needs with our own is one of the most critical of self-regulation skills. It's a very important aspect of children's social play with peers (see 'Team play' in Chapter 2), where they're intrinsically motivated to discover the rewards of cooperation, turn-taking and other rule-based behaviour. But cooperation isn't the same as compliance, and obedient imitation of adult behaviour doesn't necessarily lead to deeper learning. Perhaps girls' flying start in education is based on an ability to do as they're told, to please the nice grown-ups, and to reap at a very formative age the extrinsic rewards of smiles, ticks and pats on the head.

Good girls and naughty boys

The female of the species does seem to be more naturally adapted to people-pleasing. One research study showed that, by the age of one, girls look to their carers for signs of approval four times more often than boys. This desire for adult endorsement could well have negative consequences for intrinsically motivated learning, since pleasing an adult carer might become at least as important as the personal satisfaction of rising to a challenge. There's therefore a good chance that girls will be more inclined than boys to avoid the sorts of messy, exploratory and risky play that adults don't usually understand (and frequently prefer to stop) but which – as indicated in Chapter 2 – bring many developmental advantages.

What's more, given the tendency of many adults towards gender stereotyping, expectations of girls may be influenced by the traditional assumption that females are 'the weaker sex'. Studies show that carers who unconsciously pass on this message deter girls from active physical play – even though, when free from adult supervision, they're at least as physically confident as boys of the same age. And once a girl's absorbed the message, she's unlikely to engage in the sorts of risky play through which, in the first half of the twentieth century, 'tomboys' honed the resilience to take on a male-dominated world. (As a former tomboy, I love the battle cry of Lady Allen of Hurtwood, an early supporter of adventure playgrounds: 'Better a broken bone than a broken spirit!')

'Naughty' boys, on the other hand, may seek (and attract) less overt adult approval but, due to that unconscious gender stereotyping, adult carers generally tolerate traditionally boyish activity during early childhood. Sometimes, in fact, they actively encourage outdated stereotypes. Some adult carers (especially male ones) are worried by perfectly natural indications of shaky gender identity in the early years so they steer their small male charges towards a distinctly macho image – these days often involving screen-based activity – thus discouraging the development of emotional sensitivity and empathy.

But if little boys have the freedom to actively explore the *real* world, many of the 'boyish' characteristics this develops, such as physical confidence, initiative and willingness to take risks can come in handy throughout life, so early exploratory learning probably gives them an edge over girls in the career stakes once schooling is over. I suspect general acceptance of a 'boyish' desire for self-determination also renders adult males less willing than their female partners to take a career break for child-rearing purposes. If sexual equality is ever to be achieved, both men and women have to acknowledge that their personal role in raising the next generation is as important (and can be at least as fulfilling) as their economic role in the workplace.

In countries with a kindergarten stage, well-attuned, well-trained practitioners have time and space to support children in learning through real play, while encouraging them to think of themselves as *people* first, 'boys' or 'girls' second. In three or four years of kindergarten education, there's time to help girls see the attractions of active, exploratory activities that build physical self-confidence, adaptability and resilience. And there's time for boys to develop, through their own self-chosen play, the social and communication skills underpinning success at school, while sensitive practitioners nurture the emotional strengths that are no less natural for males than for females. As the psychologist Cordelia Fine says in her book *The Gender Delusion*, 'Our minds, society and neurosexism[12] create difference. Together they wire gender. But the wiring is soft, not hard. It is flexible, malleable and changeable. And, if we believe this, it will continue to unravel.'

Unravelling the gender wires through play

The speed with which gender roles have changed over the last half century suggests that Fine is right. But there's still a way to go before women are genuinely equal with men in the workplace and before the responsibilities of parenting are genuinely shared between the sexes. And – since children's early experiences have a profound effect on their adult attitudes and behaviour – there's good reason for concern about the current state of play in countries where formal learning starts at a very early age.

Since play is a natural learning drive that doesn't differentiate between the sexes, equal access to the types of 'real play' described in Chapter 2 should help unravel some of the neurological wiring that traps boys and girls in stereotypical gender roles. Yet from the age of three, the play available to children is now mainly:

- highly gendered 'junk play' at home, which transforms them into prettified princesses or edgy superheroes
- adult-directed play at pre-school, where all-too-often the princesses demonstrate their capacity to be 'good', while the superheroes check out how often they can be 'naughty'.

---

12 Fine's term for the use of neuroscientific research to support pre-existing ideas of inherent sex differences.

And once children are four or five, play is supplanted for a good part of the day by the need to knuckle down to the three Rs. Many 'naughty' boys are then disadvantaged in the education system because they haven't managed to cope with such an early start; while the 'good' girls are disadvantaged later, in the world of work, because they *did* manage to cope with it. Rather than unravelling the stereotypical strands, an early-start policy merely tightens the knots, with damaging consequences for both sexes.

To mitigate the effects of market-driven gender stereotyping, we should be giving boys and girls plenty of time to develop as individuals through real play in a screen-free environment – as often as possible outdoors, where active, creative play comes naturally to children. They need time and space to discover their own strengths, and sensitive adult support to help them overcome any developmental weaknesses, including gender-stereotypical ones, for example:

Boys	Girls
Time for developing the social and language skills required for school-based learning, through play with other children and interactions with supportive adults.	Time for self-chosen, personally directed, intrinsically motivating play, to counter-balance any tendency towards over-compliance and 'people pleasing'.
The opportunity to indulge in active, outdoor play, to hone physical coordination and control, and thus develop their overall powers of self-regulation.	Support and encouragement to engage in active outdoor play, to increase physical self-confidence, emotional resilience and the 'can-do' attitude they'll one day need to succeed in the workplace

Boys	Girls
Opportunities to engage in self-directed extended play and creative, open-ended activities that develop the capacity to focus and sustain their attention, and to collaborate with others towards a shared goal.	Encouragement to develop the personal initiative, self-confidence, risk-taking and problem-solving skills they'll need at work, through self-directed extended play and creative, open-ended activities.
Time to develop the physical, social and emotional maturity required for school-based learning.	Time to realise their own potential as learners, rather than relying on adult direction from a very early age.
Time to develop the empathy they'll need when they become parents themselves, through the support and example of adult carers who are highly attuned to children's individual developmental needs.	Opportunities, through social play and the example of adult carers, to recognise that caring for (and about) others is not just a matter of 'people-pleasing', but an essential human quality, as necessary for survival as physical skills.

These are the sort of experiences that a high-quality kindergarten stage can provide. What's more, they also promote mental and physical health. Three to four years in a co-educational, play-based kindergarten should help boys to get the most out of school, girls to flourish in the workplace, and both sexes to become caring adults and committed lifelong learners.

***

Every year, the World Economic Forum compiles a Global Gender Gap index, measuring female economic participation, education, health and political empowerment. In 2015 the top four countries were – guess who? – Iceland, Norway, Finland and Sweden. (The UK was number 18 and the USA 28.) It seems that the Nordic countries' record in terms of sexual equality is as impressive as that for economic equality. They must be doing something right.

In the next chapter, I look in more detail at the most educationally successful of the Nordic countries over recent years – Finland. And I argue that its enviable record of economic prosperity, gender equality *and* social justice has been largely achieved by the way it cares for all its children… boys and girls, rich and poor.

Chapter 6
FINNISH FOUNDATIONS

Why Finland lets children play till they're seven, how this has contributed to the country's educational success... and why it also helps create a 'good society'

'How did your country get such a wonderful kindergarten system?' I asked the politician.

It was 2004 and I was in Finland for the *Times Educational Supplement* to find out why they came top of all the international surveys for literacy. Given my new-found interest in child development, it hadn't taken long to work out that the Finnish early years policy was clearly implicated.

The politician was blond, about fortyish, with a serious Scandinavian face and an unpronounceable name I've long since forgotten. But I'll never forget his answer. 'It was not always like this,' he said carefully. 'Thirty years ago we thought: "How do we get a good society?" And we said: "We must look after our little children."'

Right from the start

I've since discovered that he was referring to the Finnish childcare crisis, which happened in the 1970s, twenty years earlier than in the UK. With children at home till the age of seven, a serious lack of out-of-home childcare and a great many mothers clamouring to go out to work, politicians clearly had to get involved. Like the other Nordic nations, the Finns have a deep-seated commitment to publicly funded services, so, in pursuit of a 'good society', the government began a steady expansion of state-subsidised day care facilities for children aged between three and seven.

Over the next twenty years they built up a network of local authority day care centres and by the mid-1990s they'd extended the state subsidy to cover the under-threes, with the option of a 'home care' allowance for parents who prefer to look after their own babies and toddlers. This was accompanied by a gradual extension of maternity and paternity leave (which now adds up to about a year and is covered by generous state benefits, linked to income) and legislation to develop family-friendly working practices.

In 2005, the Finnish system of childcare was singled out for special praise in an international survey by the OECD as 'a continuum of support for parents until children are in their teens... flexible parental leave, high quality childcare and reduced working hours for parents of young children.' Which just shows what politicians can do if they put their mind to it.

When I revisited Finland in 2015 on a research trip for *Upstart*, my first conversation about early years education was with a waiter at the hotel, who turned out to hail from Yorkshire. He told me enthusiastically about the support his family received from the moment his Finnish wife found she was pregnant, including the 'Baby Box' that appeared when his son was born[13] and the day care centre he now attends. 'The staff,' he said, 'are fabulous!'

---

13 All babies born in Finland are registered for a Baby Box when their mother attends her first ante-natal check up. When the baby is born she receives a sturdy cardboard box, containing everything needed for the first couple of months, such as nappies, other baby products and clothes (including outdoor clothing). It also contains a mattress which can be put inside the box, turning it into a cradle. The message is that successful parenthood isn't about spending money.

Charges for this early education and care vary, depending on income and the number of children in a family (it's free to the poorest families) but they're modest compared to those in the USA or UK because parental contributions make up only about 15 per cent of the overall costs. The remaining 85 per cent, which includes the midday meals, is down to taxpayers. Income tax rates (including both national and municipal taxes) are higher than in many western countries but the Finns are generally happy to pay for their excellent education, health and other social services because they enhance the quality of everyone's lives. These are the responsibility of the municipalities (the 320 self-governing areas into which Finland is divided, some of which are cities or towns), so the politicians involved are highly accountable to local people.

No country is perfect, of course, but Finland is always high on the World Happiness Index and has an enviable record in surveys of many social factors, including, as mentioned earlier in this book:

- consistently low levels of poverty and crime
- consistently high levels of equality, education, health and wellbeing.

In 2012, a survey found they also have the lowest level of family breakdown in Europe. Perhaps that's because, as research is now showing, people who've had a happy, secure childhood tend to forge stronger personal relationships as adults. On the whole, forty years after deciding to do the best for their little children, they seem to have achieved a pretty good society.

However, the world moves on and Finland's challenge now is to keep that society in good shape for the next forty years. Like all countries, they face financial pressures due to the worldwide economic downturn, so the charges for early education and care are set to rise for all income groups, the adult-child daycare ratio for the over-threes will soon be raised to 1:8 and entitlement may be reduced to twenty hours a week for families where one parent is at home. There's also widespread concern, in a country unused to immigration, about the economic and social problems that may accompany the integration of families from less fortunate parts of the world into Finnish society.

Not surprisingly, during my 2015 visit I sensed anxiety among early years and social work professionals that wasn't there a decade earlier. So I was very interested to find out whether the Finns are still managing to keep things right from the start for their little children. I wasn't disappointed.

Time and space to play

'Our feeling is that we want a child to be a child as long as he wants to be,' says Hannu Kahapää, the director of Kaivopuisto Day Care Centre in central Helsinki, as we watch thirty-odd three to six year olds playing out in the spring sunshine. It's a national habit in all the Nordic countries to get out and about as often as possible because the long, dark winters mean people really value the sunlight. This has meant Nordic children have always had the many benefits of outdoor play outlined in Chapter 2. Today, Hannu tells us, this batch will be outdoors most of the morning. 'We can do everything outside that we do inside,' he says.

This playground is pretty basic compared to some Finnish kindergartens I've seen – it doesn't have a wooded area, a garden or a paddling pool, for instance. But it does have a climbing frame with rope ladders and slide, several swings, two sandpits, a collection of bikes and trikes... and an awful lot of space. I reflect ruefully that, in UK inner cities, school playgrounds of this size often cater for ten times as many small active bodies. Space is essential for every sort of play.

As well as Hannu, my guide Kaisu Muuronen[14] and me, there are quite a few other adults watching these children. The adult:child

---

14 I met Kaisu Muuronen, who organised the visits for my research trip, through the World Organisation for Early Childhood Education. She also came along each day, to act as guide and translator, and I'll never be able to thank her enough.

ratio for three to seven year olds in fulll-time day care in Finland is currently 1:7 – one early years teacher and two other practitioners for every 21 children – so there's plenty of opportunity for day care staff to get to know their charges well. The atmosphere is relaxed and informal – when I do a quick inventory, one of the adults is chatting to children as she pushes them on the swings, two are deep in conversation with a little group in a sandpit, another keeps an eye on some boys balancing on the climbing frame and a fifth is observing a gaggle of girls involved in some sort of pretend play.

I ask about planning and objectives for the session and Hannu looks disdainful. 'Educational objectives are for teachers, not for children,' he says, recognising that, as a visitor from the UK, I'm referring to the sort of explicit learning targets our children are often expected to pursue. He explains that planning is minimal although, as of this year, all children must have a personal plan for education and care, negotiated with their parents. These plans become particularly important if practitioners have any concerns about a particular child, in which case the centre immediately contacts the parents to work out the best way forward and, if necessary, brings in specialist assistance. The idea is to sort any out problems as quickly as possible, before they develop into anything more serious – and hopefully before the child starts school. Otherwise the practitioners' role is to support children's play and sometimes, in true Vygotskyan fashion, to help extend their learning as developmentally appropriate to each individual.

'We identify a child's level of understanding then help move forward,' Hannu says.

'Seize the moment!' adds Kaisu and he nods sagely.

For the same reason, record-keeping is also minimal: 'We don't do tick lists, individual files or portfolios. We trust the play. I want my staff to be with the children or talking about the children, not doing paperwork.' Parents are kept in touch with what goes on by an email newsletter once a week, informal chats with the staff when dropping off or picking up their children, and one or two official parent-teacher meetings per year.

The centre also shares a couple of iPads with three other settings, and every few weeks a member of staff makes snatches of video to share with mums and dads. 'Parents like to see what their children have been up to, so we film group activities and children's play. It can also be a help if parents have a worry. If a child is crying when his mother leaves, the video can show how soon he settles down – that's reassuring for her.'

I think of children this age back in the UK, where the focus is on 'school readiness' till four or five, then the three Rs for five and six year olds, and where children's progress is meticulously plotted and recorded. How would the average English parent – accustomed to tests, targets, objectives, goals, tick-lists, profiles and endless record-keeping – react to the laid-back attitude of Hannu and his staff, as they watch the children play and wait patiently to 'seize the moment'? Could they ever recognise the professionalism that goes into this sort of developmentally appropriate practice?

Then I remember that my Yorkshire waiter thinks his son's Finnish day care staff are 'fabulous'.

A tale of two systems

There are many ways in which Finnish kindergartens seem 'fabulous' to me, compared with the UK version. One is the nationally decreed ratio of carers to children, which in England is 13:1 for the over-threes, meaning that an English practitioner has responsibility for almost twice as many children as her Finnish counterpart. A second is the national curriculum followed by early years staff in each country. In England, the Early Years Foundation Stage framework is a detailed description of what's to be covered in six subject areas, and long lists of the expected attainment levels for children at each stage of the system. It's probably as top-down a document for this stage of education as it's possible to imagine.

In contrast, Finland's Curriculum for Early Childhood Education and Care (ECEC) has no mention of what children are expected to attain, just general principles, such as:

> The primary concern is to support development of each child's positive self-concept and healthy self-esteem and to ensure equal membership of the group. Schoolwork should be playful and involve action-based group and individual guidance stemming from children's development level. It should promote children's cognitive, in particular linguistic, as well as socio-emotional development and their ability to learn new things and also prevent learning difficulties.[15]

Goals in Finland are, as Hannu said, for adults, not children. ECEC practitioners are trusted to achieve their personal goals as educators by providing a warm, supportive environment in which children can regularly experience 'the joy of learning'. Sometimes this may involve 'seizing the moment', at other times it might mean backing off. The choice depends on informed, attuned, on-the-spot decision-making.

For this reason, Finland takes pains to ensure its ECEC practitioners are as well-informed about child development as possible. At least a third of the staff in any kindergarten must have degrees in early childhood education, and many hold masters degrees involving five years study (this includes all pre-primary teachers working on school premises because all Finnish primary school teachers must be qualified to masters level). In fact, the proportion of highly qualified staff in kindergartens is often far higher than the prescribed minimum, partly because ECEC staff are highly respected and partly because it's such a fulfilling job. Hannu has a masters degree, many of his staff are university

---

15 The ECEC curriculum in Finland is currently under review, as the final stage in a revision of the entire educational system, most of which is now in place. The new version is due to be finalised by the end of 2016 but the overall ethos seems unlikely to change.

graduates and others, whom he calls 'nurses', have completed three-year polytechnic ECEC degrees. Practitioners' education is also on-going, with an annual in-service programme provided by their municipality's education department.

The contrast with England is stark. Some practitioners have specialist early years degrees or nursery nursing certificates, but many nursery staff have minimal qualifications and others are trained for primary, not early years, education. I remember an interesting conversation with a nursery nurse, whose nursery chain had employed a primary teacher to fulfil government requirements for qualified staff. However, she 'hadn't the first idea how to be with little kids' so was now in an office devising project-based learning activities for the five nurseries. She toiled away at this all day and the nursery nurses shoved the resulting documentation in a drawer because 'it just isn't right for the children and anyway we've got the EYFS for that'. I dread to think what her irrelevant qualification was costing the nursery (and, indeed, the fee-paying parents).

In 2012, recommendations for improving English early years training and qualifications were welcomed by the profession but the main suggestions were subsequently ignored by the government that had commissioned them. It seemed they too work on the principle that 'we've got the EYFS for that'. So, rather than training up the Early Years workforce, then trusting them to make informed on-the-spot decisions, they prefer to rely on a heavily prescribed national curriculum, top-down targets and an educational culture of fear.

The difference in ethos continues throughout the two educational systems: in the UK, a tests-and-targets agenda keeps everyone on government-determined tramlines, while Finland simply trusts everyone to learn. There's no standardised testing until students matriculate at age 18 or 19, school inspections were abandoned in the early 1990s, and the guidance provided to teachers and carers – at both national and municipal level – is referred to as 'steering by information' (i.e. early years experts provide evidence-based information and professionals decide how, and even whether, to use it in their own establishment).

Finland's hands-off approach achieves far better results than England's control-freakery. Maybe that's because the aim of Finnish education is to help all children reach their full potential as *autonomous* learners. When everyone in a system is intrinsically motivated, there's no need for heavy-handed, top-down direction. And there's a much greater chance of genuine, meaningful learning.

Indoor time and space

After our sojourn in the Helsinki playground Kaisu and I are given a tour of the building. Some Finnish day care centres are purpose-built with every imaginable mod con, but this centre, like many UK pre-school settings, is a converted early twentieth-century building that was once a large family home. Nevertheless, my overwhelming impression is still one of time and space to play.

Most UK nurseries I visit feel cluttered – furniture and toys clog up the rooms, every inch of wall space is covered in posters, charts and pictures… often there's even stuff hanging from the ceiling. It's as though the practitioners are trying to prove how busy everyone is, how much the children are learning, how *stimulating* nursery can be. But here equipment is stashed out of sight when not in use (there are lots of storage units in typically blond Scandinavian wood) and – apart from an alphabet chart, some children's artwork and a few pictures and labels – the walls are bare. The space in this building is clearly meant to be filled with play, not stuff. And, since everyone trusts the play to come from the children, there's no need for copious visual evidence of adult endeavour.

It seems that Finnish practitioners recognise that the last thing children need these days is more artificial 'stimulation' – in a fast-moving, high-tech culture, the brains of twenty-first-century babies, toddlers and pre-schoolers are often relentlessly *over*-stimulated from dawn to dusk. So rather than add to this frenzy, a Finnish kindergarten is an oasis of calm, where young minds can develop at their own speed. When Kaisu and I visit the Helsinki Education

Department next day, we're shown a film – *Premises and Pedagogy* – in which local practitioners share ideas on using space productively, keeping noise-levels down and reducing clutter. Copies have been sent out to all the settings in the municipality so that good ideas can be stirred around the profession.[16]

In the Kaivopuisto Day Care Centre, the little children (0–3 years) inhabit the first floor – a number of small, comfortable rooms with a home-like feel, including a bedroom for napping after lunch. The ratio of staff to children is 1:4, as in the UK, and my quick inventory of adult activity reveals two practitioners playing with groups of children, one reading a story to a little girl on her lap while a toddler clings on to her leg, and another helping a child make handprints. It doesn't seem much different from the baby/toddler rooms in UK nurseries I visit, except that there are fewer children here and the age groups are mixed, giving the impression of a large extended family. Like most Finns, local parents clearly make use of their year's parental leave and many claim the home-care allowance for at least part of the following two years.

The ground floor is the territory of the over-threes. It has several rooms for group activities (which this afternoon will be making cards and presents for Mother's Day next Sunday) and a large hall for games and active play. There's a huge painting of a pirate ship on the hall wall, the backdrop for a pirate theme the children have chosen for this half-term. When the proto-pirates finally come in from the playground after three hours in the open air, a male teacher brings a group into the hall for half an hour of songs, games and chat.

They're clearly following the centre's 'curriculum', which Hannu described when Kaisu and I arrived. It was delightfully brief: 'Every morning we must do outdoor activities, free play, singing and games.' The final game this morning involves the children lying in a circle on the floor while, amid much giggling, the teacher counts their feet –

16 One simple idea I spotted was the numbers 1 to 20 stencilled on a stone staircase, so children could see them and count as they ascended. When I got home, I did my own bit of stirring by mentioning this to a UK early years resources supplier.

Kaisu explains that it's a 'dipping' game to choose the order in which they'll go off to lunch.

As in every Finnish kindergarten I've visited, this meal is a civilised affair with flowers on the tables and nutritious, locally sourced food. Staff and children eat together, providing an opportunity for more conversation and the development of table manners. After they've eaten, it's Quiet Time and the children can choose either to take a nap or listen to stories. Most choose the latter, though some of the older ones prefer to read for themselves. In the afternoon, it's off outside to play again.

Caring communities

It's not just the parents of Finnish under-threes who often choose not to send their children to day care. Despite the excellent facilities and generous subsidies, some mums and dads prefer to care full-time for their three- to six-year-old children at home too, and many send them to the centre only some days a week. Even children who are enrolled full-time sometimes don't turn up – perhaps one parent has the day off or granny has come to stay for a while and the children want to spend time with her.

This presents no problem, since practitioners know the importance of family time, especially when children are young and it's helping build the strong relationships between generations upon which authoritative parenting depends. At Hannu Kahapää's centres it's therefore also taken for granted that parents and children can arrive at any time in the morning and collect them early if they wish. The come-and-go-as-you-please policy means there's a delightfully informal quality to parent–staff interactions.

To start with, though, I witnessed the casual comings and goings in amazement, because subsidised attendance for three to five year olds at English pre-schools assumes regular attendance. Under the terms of the Common Inspection Framework, all out-of-home carers, including childminders, are expected to monitor, report and explain absences. Repeated non-attendance or partial attendance (including absence for a family holiday during term-time) soon lands parents in hot water with the educational authorities. Basically, while Finnish ECEC is genuinely seen as a shared enterprise between parents and professionals, English politicians' obsession with accelerating academic progress means any time away from the eagle-eye of EYFS practitioners could lead to pre-schoolers being 'left behind' in their educational rat-race.

There's a huge amount of research showing that good parent–teacher relationships are extremely important throughout the educational process, and at this early stage it's vital to nurture the relationship between parents and professional carers. Insistence on regular attendance *before* compulsory school age gives the impression that families aren't trusted to raise their own offspring, thus making genuine partnership difficult. It also disempowers parents and adds to an already teetering mountain of bureaucracy for practitioners. On the other hand, Finland's more laid-back approach creates a climate of trust and in which every day centre is also seen as a community resource, a trusted source of information about early child development.

Later in my trip, I saw how this principle also applies to other aspects of out-of-school care. I was taken to visit a 'playground centre' where seven to ten year olds can go for after-school care if their parents can't collect them at the end of the school day (the over-tens go to a youth centre nearby). The playground concerned has a wide variety of outdoor facilities (including a paddling pool) and many adult helpers to lead organised activities and keep an eye on children while they play. It also has a two full-time professional child-care workers, based in the 'Family House' where children go for snacks and indoor relaxation (no TV in there, but plenty of books, games and a piano for musical activities). During the day, this Family House is used for community events, including meetings and clubs for parents, designed to help them provide developmentally appropriate support for children under ten.

Nevertheless, Finland – like the rest of the twenty-first-century global village – is subject to cultural change. In recent years, Finnish families have spent increasing amounts of time gazing at screens, meaning that many of the day-to-day activities through which children's development was once naturally nurtured are dying out. This includes the sort of experiences which, back in Chapter 4, were listed as creating 'lucky' children, who find learning to read, write and reckon comes 'naturally'.

This is one of the reasons why, in 2015, Finland changed its attitude to attendance for the final year of kindergarten. All six-year-old children are now required to attend 700 hours of free 'pre-primary education' a year (that is, every morning, five days a week) either in a day care centre or a primary pre-school class. However, while this effectively lowers the starting age for compulsory education, it's been made very clear that the pre-primary year is *not* formal schooling. As has always been the case, the ethos is still essentially play-based, following the simple curriculum Hannu outlined, but with slightly more attention to activities that develop the underpinning skills of literacy and numeracy. In most pre-primary classes, this means two teacher-directed sessions per day, each lasting around half an hour.

Now we are six

A couple of days after the day care centre visit, Kaisu and I turn up at a Helsinki primary school to see what pre-primary reading and writing involves. On this occasion, we're accompanied by Maria Kay, an email acquaintance of mine who's researching a PhD on the relationship between music and literacy. There's been surprisingly little research so far on this subject so she wants to see what exactly Finland does that impacts so favourably on their literacy results.

The primary school is in a twentieth-century building in a built-up area of Helsinki – very similar to inner city schools in the UK – which means six year olds here are shorter on indoor space than those in day care centres. Nevertheless, the practitioners have done their best, keeping all the furniture at the edges of the room, and when we arrive the children are sitting with their teacher in the middle of an empty floor, talking. She's provided us with a short summary of her 'Lesson for Linguistic Skills' (see Appendix 6 – the 'sportive play' it describes turns out to involve a great deal of hopping). As someone whose main interests in life are child development, linguistics and literacy, I settle down to enjoy myself.

The session starts with a discussion about feelings, linked to the characters in a puppet village the children have created (I spot their puppet tree-house village on a wall display). This chat leads them to compose a party invitation to cheer up a lonely puppet, the teacher scribing as they tell her what to write. The group then splits up so they all get a shot at three games: 'sportive' hopping around common syllables on the floor; a card game in the corner for grammar (those fiendishly tricky Finnish word-endings), and some interesting gymnastics as pupils are challenged to make letter-shapes with their bodies (the children who can write are helped to compose their own sentences for the party invitation on a whiteboard).

There's no evidence of boredom among those six year olds (mostly girls) who are obviously already competent readers and writers. I do note, however, that these children enjoy helping their peers during the group activities. At the end of the lesson, they happily join in with the rest of the class in various sorts of free play, during which some children choose to work on the ubiquitous Mothers Day cards. Throughout the Finnish education system, all lessons are followed by a break – which younger children take in the open air if possible.[17]

As we're ushered out of the pre-primary class to see a primary lesson, I'm feeling as impressed as I was ten years earlier when Agneta introduced me to Finnish kindergarten practice (see Chapter 4). What I've just seen reaffirms my conviction that we could teach little children everything they need to know

---

17 A typical lesson for primary children would be forty-five minutes long, followed by a fifteen minute break. However, depending on what they are doing, the teacher may run two lessons together and give a slightly longer break afterwards.

about phonics and grammar through fun and games, without subjecting them to tedious drill or written exercises. What's more, all the physical activity in the 'Lesson for Linguistic Skills' has contributed to the children's embodied understanding of symbolic systems, and their animated discussion to their language and listening skills. And, since this sort of 'lesson' is intrinsically motivating, the children *want* to go on learning – as we're led off to view a Grade One primary literacy lesson, I notice a group who've chosen to carry on with the grammar card game during their free play and one little boy painstakingly writing a message in his mum's card.

Another quote from Hannu Kahapää comes to mind: 'Keep the children at the centre. They like to play. They are happy to wait for school – they like to play.' Why can't politicians in my own country see that playful activity is the best way to prepare young children for learning, literacy and life?

Patterns and sounds

Maria, on the other hand, is looking anxious. It's not until we've seen the seven year olds' literacy session and are heading to the headmaster's office for a talk about the school's philosophy that I realise why. There was no music in the Lesson for Language and Literacy Skills or the one we've just seen. Considering she's come to Finland on the strength of an article I wrote raving about the use of music in early years, I begin to feel a little worried too.

The headteacher launches into a talk about the pre-primary class. The state pays for children's attendance at school between 8.30 a.m. and 12.30 p.m, and then for their lunch, but if parents want them to stay for the afternoon there's a fee. However, it's pretty modest – between 0 and 120 euro (about £85) a week – so most children do a full day in his school. He goes through the areas listed in the National Curriculum for Pre-Primary Education that practitioners must bear in mind when working with the children: language and interaction; maths, ethics and outlook on life; environmental and natural sciences; health; development of physical skills; art and culture. He tells us yet again that the children learn by playing, experimenting, exploring and inquiring, in interaction with other children and adults.

Not only is all this now pretty familiar, I'm also feeling increasingly cross that my home country is so far back in the dark ages in terms of early years education. So I distract myself by scrutinising a portrait of a gloomy-looking man, with a bald head and piercing Nordic eyes, that's strategically placed above the headteacher's desk. Who is he? The school's founder? A famous Finnish educator? The head's granddad? The portrait fixes me with a mournful gaze as the headmaster explains arrangements for transition from pre-primary to primary school, and Maria prepares to attack.

When he pauses for breath, she lobs in a question: 'Does music play an important role in the school?'

Like many primary heads I've known, he seems surprised to be interrupted. But then he smiles and gives Maria a tolerant but old-fashioned look – similar to the one I received from Agneta a decade ago when I asked 'Why do you do so much music?' (see 'Let's hear it for story and song!' in Chapter 4).

'Yes, of course,' he replies. 'Would you like to see the music room?' As he ushers us out of the room to visit it, I duck over to read the label on the portrait. It's Sibelius.

Maria practically swoons at the primary school's music room, which has racks of guitars, violins, and wind instruments on the walls, a piano, keyboard and drum kit. The school's specialist music teacher is in there, tidying up after a lesson. This lady is clearly kept pretty busy, running singing sessions for every class, teaching all the seven year olds to play the recorder and supervising tuition in a variety of other instruments for children who want to learn. As Maria bombards her with questions, I learn with interest that all Finnish early years practitioners must take music courses and most can play an instrument themselves.

Yes, of course music plays an important role in Finnish kindergarten and primary education. It's so important that no one had thought it necessary to mention it to us. In the land of Sibelius, everyone clearly takes it for granted that 'music trains the mind to pattern and the ears to sound.'

Talking teaching

My only disappointment in visiting Helsinki kindergartens, as opposed to those I saw a decade earlier in the more rural town of Espoo, is that they don't have such exciting playgrounds. The Espoo children had constant access to green spaces, with trees, grass and rocks to romp on. However, Maria and I are reassured about this at a meeting with Satu Järvenkallas, Helsinki's Director of Early Education and Care, and Arja-Sisko Holappa, who's in charge of the pre-primary year for the National Finnish Board of Education.

One of the messages they want us to carry away is the importance of 'opening doors to the outdoors' and ensuring that city children get out of the classroom as often as possible and discover local amenities such as museums and Helsinki Zoo. Above all, kindergarten teachers are encouraged to take children on regular trips into the local countryside. It is Satu who shows us the *Premises and Pedagogy* video (practitioners sharing ways of improving their practice indoors and out), which includes tips about about organising visits to the woods such as:

When you arrive, give the children at least half an hour just to explore.

Go back to familiar places where they can pick up the play from last time and feel safe to explore. You need at least two hours in the woods.

It doesn't matter what the weather's like. Being out in the rain makes children sleep better!

Watching this film sparks a chat about the pedagogical advantages of the outdoors – from developing children's problem-solving strategies and understanding of scientific principles, to all the different opportunities for counting: 'You can count stones, trees, steps... jumps!' As in every conversation I've ever had with early years educators – not just in Finland, but everywhere, including the UK – there's real excitement when we start swapping stories about children's natural potential for learning.

Then I remember why I'm there. 'English practitioners know all this stuff too,' I say glumly. 'They just don't get anywhere near enough time and freedom to put it into practice. Children have two years in nursery at the most, and much of the staff's time is taken up with planning, assessment and record-keeping. You should see the risk assessment forms they have to complete before they go on any sort of excursion!'

'Yes,' says Maria, 'In a way, it hurts to see how you do things here. The teachers back home are just so ground down by the system.'

'But practitioners' enthusiasm and commitment is vital!' cries Arja-Sisko, and this time we Brits do the old-fashioned looks.

'It *was* more like this in the UK in the olden days,' I reminisce. 'When I was a primary teacher in the 1980s, you could take kids out to explore the local area whenever you wanted. And it was such good fun thinking up new ideas and making materials that I'd be often be up doing it till midnight.'

'Put that in your book!' says Satu. So I have.

What? Even the Finns?

Then Satu astonishes me, producing a quote as memorable as the one with which I opened this chapter. 'I'm not sure,' she says, 'that we appreciate as a nation how much our early years policy contributes to the good results.'

What? Even the Finns don't recognise the importance of professional early years practice in laying sound foundations for school-based learning? The country where politicians put their money where their mouth is, and *really* try to do their best for their little children? The country with the most highly educated early years workforce in the world? I sit blinking for a moment, trying to digest this idea. Since Finland has developed an early years system that sends almost every child to primary school bright-eyed, bushy-tailed and ready to learn, I'd somehow assumed that all Finns understood the significance of what happens in kindergartens... but...

Satu is looking at me kindly.

'Oh gosh, Pasi Sahlberg's book...,' I stutter, and she gives an inscrutable smile.

Pasi Sahlberg – the international authority on Finland's educational success – is currently wowing audiences in the USA. When I read his 2012 book *Finnish Lessons*, I noticed that he scarcely mentioned early years but soon forgot the omission due to excitement about his description of Finland's egalitarian educational ethos – 'Equity first' – and the trust his country puts in teachers to assess and direct children's progress. As Sahlberg says in an article on the Stanford University website,

> Education has always been an integral part of Finnish culture and teachers currently enjoy great respect and trust in Finland. Finns regard teaching as a noble, prestigious profession – akin to medicine, law, or economics – and one driven by moral purpose rather than material interests.

Since any teacher is entitled to be wowed by that thought, I forgive myself for forgetting what scant attention he paid to early years.

And indeed, the Finnish school system and its well-educated and well-respected workforce are entitled to be extremely proud of their achievements. But I wonder if they'd have achieved anywhere near as much if their children's natural capacity to learn hadn't already been nurtured by a highly qualified early years workforce? Or, indeed, whether that workforce would be anywhere near as effective if Finland didn't have such a late school starting age and a long-established cultural attachment to three critically important elements of early years education – language and listening skills, music and outdoor play?

Warning Bells

Over the last couple of years, Finland has been revising its national curriculum, so this meeting is also an opportunity to hear more about the framework for the pre-primary year from Arja-Sisko Holappa and new guidance on media education from Saara Pääjärvi of the National Audiovisual Institute. Both presentations are excellent. However, now that I've realised the Finnish educational establishment is not actually perfect, a tiny worm of anxiety has begun to wriggle at the back of my brain.

Arja-Sisko's pre-primary framework is, rightly, concerned with 'active, context-based learning'. She tells us that primary teaching in the past has been 'a little bit boring', so the principles underpinning kindergarten education are henceforth also to be applied throughout primary schooling. While all in favour of activity and exciting contexts for seven to eleven year olds' learning, I have miserable memories of what happened in the UK back in the 1970s and 80s when war broke out between traditional and progressive educational theorists (see Chapter 1).

It occurs to me that the Grade 1 literacy lesson I saw a decade ago in Espoo couldn't have been more different from the one Maria and I watched the previous day in a Helsinki primary school. The seven year olds in Espoo sat silently writing in their exercise books for half an hour, with a brief break for an action song about syllabification. They seemed quite content to apply themselves to their written task and the lesson would've gladdened any traditionalist heart. Yesterday's lesson in Helsinki was almost entirely oral, bubbling with fun and drama – the 1970s progressives would've loved it.

My experience of primary teaching is that children need *both* sorts of experience to keep them on track – the formal/academic *and* the motivating/playful. Keeping a sensitive balance isn't easy but when teaching swings too far in either direction, problems ensue. Reading and writing are old-fashioned technologies, requiring traditional methods of teaching to some extent. While primary children need the oral, motivating, progressive stuff to provide reasons for sitting down and practising their literacy skills, the practice can't be entirely sacrificed to the fun. It was when UK teachers were seduced into losing this balance that 1980 traditionalists were able to blow the progressives out of the water, leading to the grim state of affairs in England today.

One of the reasons I so admire Finnish kindergartens is that they ensure the vast majority of seven year olds arrive in primary school with sufficient self-regulation skills to tackle the formal, academic, traditional elements of literacy learning. As Ofsted commented in 2004, their boredom threshold is much higher than UK children. It would be tragic if Finnish primary teachers become so pre-occupied with 'active, context-based learning' that they forget to keep nurturing those powers of self-regulation.

I'm sure Finnish educational gurus are well aware of the need for balance – this is certainly one of the most balanced nations I've come across. Nevertheless, I left Helsinki wondering what would happen to Finland's international status if the new primary curriculum inadvertently tips teachers too far in a 'progressive' direction.

Old and new literacies

Another tiny warning bell sounded during the presentation on media education, in which Saara Pääjärvi explained that children growing up in a multimedia world need to understand all kinds of communications media, including digital technology, so schools mustn't be 'media-free bubbles'. While I wouldn't quibble with any of the points she made, I fervently hope Finland doesn't change its current – very sensible and balanced – attitude to new technology in the kindergarten and early primary years.

Finnish children are supported in developing their communication skills via a wide variety of media but on neither of my visits did I see any 'screen-based teaching' in the settings and classrooms I visited – apparently, they do now have the odd interactive whiteboard, but these are tucked away in special rooms for occasional use. The primary teachers in Espoo and Helsinki shared words and pictures with their classes via a visualiser, a machine that projects an enlarged image of anything you place on it. On the whole, young children's learning in Finland still happens in real time and real space, and is mediated by real live adults.

This is in direct contrast to UK practice, where almost every school classroom now has an interactive whiteboard (as do many nurseries), even the youngest children are encouraged to play on computers and, in recent years, tablets have been doled out liberally to children of three and over. Many of these tablets are iPads, which is deeply ironic since neither Steve Jobs nor his sidekick Johnny Ives let their own children use them. However, the marketers at Apple know that brand allegiance starts early so there have been some great deals for schools to ensure the right brand reaches the youngest children.

UK politicians fell in love with technology back in the 1990s and ring-fenced parts of every school's budget for buying in generation after generation of hard and software. Goodness knows how many extra teachers could have been employed with the millions of pounds that were wasted by this constant updating. Instead, educational suppliers mopped up the money and produced electronic 'learning packages' for everything under the sun, with the result that many under-sevens now spend hours of every school day staring at screens of various kinds.

In 2015, an OECD report that 'computers do not improve pupil results' led to the first media stirrings of concern about growing reliance on screen-based learning in UK schools, which gave some hope to the many early years practitioners who doubt the wisdom of increasing investment in technology for young children. Given the contents of Chapter 4, it will come as no surprise that I too am firmly in favour of 'keeping it real' during early childhood. Young children learn best from active, embodied experience and opportunities to talk and listen, not gazing at images and symbols on a screen. In Chapter 5, I also mention the ways children's linguistic and intellectual development are affected by watching stories on screen rather than listening to them told or read aloud by real live human beings. However, I believe there's another pressing reason to limit screen-based technology during the first seven or eight years of children's education. It's summed up by a quote from the American essayist Neil Postman in his book *The Disappearance of Childhood*: 'Print means a slowed down mind... the written and then the printed word brought a new kind of social organisation to civilisation. It brought logic, science, education, civilité.' Learning to read and write helps pass these habits of civilisation through the generations, because every child has to slow down his or her mind, thus developing the potential to think and reason better.

This isn't to say there's anything wrong with digital learning. It's just that, if children become hooked on high-tech quick-fix rewards before they're six or seven, they may not be able to slow down their minds sufficiently to acquire basic literacy skills and then build on them through practice. As Postman also said, 'electronics speeds up the brain'. So, while schools should obviously not be 'media-free bubbles', they should exercise great caution about the ways they use electronic media in the early stages. I reckon much of Finland's educational success is due to the way their kindergartens use tried-and-tested human methods of slowing down twenty-first-century children's over-stimulated brains.

Fortunately, Finland is a country that listens to its teachers. I'm sure they won't allow anything to threaten their thoughtful, professional practice. A country this clever couldn't possibly fall into any of the traps our education system tumbled into... could it?

***

It must be deeply frustrating for Finnish early years experts that their contribution to Finland's international reputation isn't properly recognised. I know kindergarten teachers believe in preparing children for life rather than for formal schooling, but when they've discovered a recipe that so resoundingly does both, they certainly deserve a round of applause from their country's educational establishment.

On the other hand, maybe Satu's inscrutable smile was a signal that they'd rather keep quiet about it. They've successfully ring-fenced their kindergarten stage as a place where children are entitled to 'learn with joy'. If academics and politicians start taking an interest in early years, they might want to start tinkering with it in all sorts of unhelpful ways, as they are doing in other western nations.

Still, I hope no international governments are converted by Pasi Sahlberg's book without first looking at Finland's pre-school practice. If they try rejigging English-speaking educational systems along the lines he suggests without first raising the school starting age and introducing a Finnish-style kindergarten stage, I fear they're doomed to abject failure. One of the reasons a tests-and-targets agenda is necessary in many western countries is that children who haven't acquired self-regulation skills need threats and rewards to keep them from running amok.

Any attempt to emulate Finland's success must to start from bottom up – providing young children with plenty of time and space to play... then patiently watching, waiting and seizing the best moments to support their natural desire to learn.

Chapter 7

CHANGING MINDS TO CHANGE THE FUTURE

Why this book was written, why early-start countries *must* change their attitude to early childhood and to the professionals who care for young children, how such a culture change can happen and why it has to start now!

She's not quite seven. Yesterday, she was messing about in the back garden, making weird horticultural mixtures in her 'mud kitchen'. Today, she's scrubbed, shining and bubbling with excitement as she arrives at primary school for the first time. The teacher welcomes her into the classroom, along with twenty-odd other boys and girls, all thrilled to be embarking on the next stage of their educational journey.

Her mum and dad are excited for her too. But they're also relieved that, so far, their daughter's childhood has been filled with the challenges of play, rather than an early start on formal schooling. She's learned the basics of reading and writing because she wanted to and she loves doing number puzzles in her head, so they're pretty sure she'll flourish at school. But her kindergarten years of outdoor adventure, music, stories, art and play have done much more than prepare her for school. Whatever the future holds, their little girl and her classmates have been as well-prepared as possible to meet it with confidence, resilience and minds of their own.

Why Upstart?

Of course, not all children who start school at seven flourish unreservedly, nor do all those who start at four or five wind up with long-term mental health problems. Countless aspects of nature and nurture influence the development of every human child, not least the love and care they receive from their families. But – given what we know about early child development and the potentially toxic effects of modern lifestyles – there's a far greater chance of educational success and long-term wellbeing if boys and girls are allowed to enjoy learning for a few years in the way young children are naturally equipped to learn.

I really enjoyed imagining that little girl in the opening paragraphs. Being towards the other end of the human life-span, I couldn't be more grateful that my own early childhood was filled with opportunities for real play, backed up by parental (and grandparental) love. Everything I've learned, both personally and professionally, in nearly seventy years has convinced me that love and play are the greatest gifts any generation can hand on to the next. Whenever and wherever we're born, every human life is inevitably filled with challenges – most of them coming completely out of the blue – and it helps a lot if the capacity for self-belief, resilience and independent thought are embedded deep in our neural networks.

Talking of unexpected challenges, I certainly didn't expect to spend the last year tapping out *Upstart*. After fifteen years of writing about child development in the modern world, I'd promised myself (and my nearest and dearest) *no more books* – it really did seem about time to follow my own advice and Get Out More. Then Fate took a hand.

In the summer of 2014, I spoke at a seminar about the role of childhood play in developing long-term resilience. A couple of early years teachers in the audience pointed out that play is now seriously threatened by the creeping schoolification of early childhood. I sought them out afterwards for a chat and we were joined by an acquaintance from the play sector, who stressed the need to revive outdoor play. We all heartily agreed that someone should Do Something About It. A week or so later, I mentioned the conversation to an editor at Floris Books and she suggested a book on the subject.

A book about the school starting age seemed the ideal way to:

- make the case for play as a vital aspect of children's health and wellbeing
- explain why putting top-down academic pressure on the under-sevens isn't just counter-productive but in some cases downright cruel
- show that other countries have found a much better way of preparing *all* children for life – and for lifelong learning.

So the plans for Getting Out More went on hold and I returned to the laptop.

Joining up the dots

However – even with a great deal of help from all the people mentioned in the Acknowledgements – putting the case together has proved more of a challenge than I expected. Apart from recent findings on 'summerborns' (see Appendix 5) there was actually very little educational research dealing specifically with the school starting age. On reflection, this is scarcely surprising. Ever since countries around the world introduced compulsory education – starting around 150 years ago – everyone's taken their own nation's starting age for granted, not least because it's enshrined in law. Mainstream educational research all round the world has therefore proceeded on the basis of each country's *status quo* and tends to be about what happens *after* formal education has begun.

Most educationists who raise the question of when formal learning should begin are early years specialists, whose voices, as mentioned in Chapter 2, are seldom heard. All of which explains why – despite mounting concern about declining educational standards, the disappearance of 'real play' from children's lives and the parlous state of the upcoming generation's mental health – neither political nor educational establishments have made the connection between these developments and an early-start policy.

Writing *Upstart* therefore involved gathering evidence from a wide range of academic disciplines – neuroscience, developmental psychology, child mental health, anthropology, sociology, evolutionary biology and the new science of wellbeing – and splicing it together with what little relevant educational research exists. Fortunately, I've had lots of practice in this sort of multi-disciplinary splicing, because it's what I've been doing ever since Sally Ward kick-started the *Toxic Childhood* research fifteen years ago. Anyway, it's meant that for the last eighteen months, I've been pulling together various pieces of evidence and attempting to join up the dots.

As I wrote, more dots kept emerging to back up the case. Perhaps the most important dots were those relating to the decline of 'real play', a subject I've been monitoring for the last twenty years. There's now no doubt whatsoever that play (especially outdoor play) is a vital factor in childhood health and wellbeing yet, despite endless reports and government policy documents, it continues to disappear from children's lives. Commercial pressures (not least the availability of sedentary screen-based entertainment at an increasingly early age) combined with adult anxieties of various kinds are squeezing play out of twenty-first-century home life. And in school and pre-school, more and more time is devoted to teacher-directed activities that supposedly develop 'school readiness'. As Professor Nancy Carlsson-Paige, a US early years expert, said in November 2015:

> Never in my wildest dreams did I think we would have to defend children's right to play... But play is disappearing from classrooms. We are seeing it shoved aside to make room for academic instruction and 'rigour'.

Another set of dots relate to increases in child and adolescent mental health problems, which, as explained in Chapter 5, often have their origins in early childhood. Although English children officially have fewer Special Educational Needs than they did in 2010 (thanks to the massaging of statistics described in Chapter 3), there's still much concern about ADHD, especially among disadvantaged children, and autistic spectrum disorder across the social classes. There have also been reports of alarming rises in self-harm, depression and eating disorders. Throughout 2015, news items kept appearing about a crisis in the UK's Child and Adolescent Mental Health Services, due to mushrooming referrals from schools, where headteachers now rate pupils' mental health as one of their most pressing concerns.

Then there are the dots relating to disadvantaged children's educational failure. In mid 2015, yet another national project was launched in the UK, with the aim of improving the literacy and numeracy skills of youngsters in the poorest sectors of society. *Read, Write, Count* is the sort of campaign to which, as a literacy specialist, I'd once have given my full support. However, writing *Upstart* has convinced me that homing in on the three Rs at an early age is likely to do more harm than good in the long run, especially for children who are already at a developmental disadvantage. Apart from anything else, it encourages politicians to get involved...

Indeed, a couple of months after the launch of *Read Write Count*, the government in my home country of Scotland announced a national drive to enhance literacy standards among disadvantaged children. It involves the introduction of standardised tests for (among others) five year olds and will almost inevitably lead to a further schoolification of early years practice. The Scottish government officials who dreamed up the idea obviously hadn't read a recent research review by the National Union of Teachers:

> There is no evidence as yet that accountability measures
> can reduce the attainment gap between disadvantaged
> pupils and their peers. There is evidence that disadvantaged
> children, who on average have lower attainment than their

peers and are therefore under greater pressure to meet targets, can become disaffected as a result of experiencing 'failure', and this is being exacerbated by recent changes to the curriculum to make it more demanding and challenging.

Meanwhile, controversy continued to rage about the baseline tests for four and five year olds introduced in 2015 in England.

The paradigm trap

The most frustrating set of dots, however, related to international statistics. In the summer of 2015, the Organisation for Economic Cooperation and Development published yet another survey of worldwide educational achievement. As usual these days, Asian countries hogged the top five places[18] but in sixth, seventh and eighth place were Finland, Estonia and Switzerland. All these countries have a school-starting age of seven and also provide a developmentally appropriate kindergarten stage for younger children. What's more, in the remaining two countries in OECD's top ten (the Netherlands and Canada) compulsory schooling begins at six and both countries take a child-centred approach to the early primary years, with no national standardised testing.

Immersed as I was in *Upstart*, I found it amazing that media coverage of the 2015 OECD survey didn't mention that the the most successful countries all had late school starting ages. In a world obsessed with number-crunching, surely that numerical

---

18 I visited Singapore, Hong Kong and Japan while working on *Toxic Childhood*, and concluded that the cultural differences between Asian countries and the Anglo-Saxon nations were so great, and child-rearing/educational practices so different, that comparisons are extremely difficult. Also, data on children's mental health, which is of particular significance in *Upstart*'s argument, isn't available for the Asian countries that top the OECD charts. (The three I visited do, however, all start formal schooling at six, while China starts at seven.)

coincidence should be flagged up by now? The late-start countries have been out-performing the rest since international comparisons began, a decade and a half ago. But then I remembered Satu Järvenkallas's comment about Finland not recognising the contribution of their early years practice to her country's academic success. I suspect that the main reason that number-crunchers are failing to join all these dots is that practically everyone, everywhere, is stuck in a classic paradigm trap.

When adults have been thoroughly schooled in the principle that *school* is where children go to learn, they automatically assume that the quality of schooling is responsible for an educational system's success or failure. It doesn't cross anyone's mind to wonder whether pre-school practice might have anything to do with it. Or how old children are when their schooling begins. Everyone just accepts that their nation's school starting age is an immutable fact of life, rather like the weather. And, anyway, how could *playing* for a couple of extra years possibly make children more successful learners?

Indeed, until fifteen years ago I was firmly trapped in this paradigm myself, and without the help of experts in early education and play, I certainly wouldn't have understood the significance of what I saw on my latest research trip to Finland. There isn't any obvious educational value in letting thirty-odd children run around having a good time, while five adults keep an eye on them. Or, indeed, in half-hour sing-along sessions, snuggling up for stories after lunch, inviting puppets to an imaginary party, playing hopping games and going on trips to the woods. They're merely the sorts of activity that 'lucky' children have always enjoyed before the serious business of schooling begins.

Nevertheless, the evidence is now beginning to emerge. As I sat tapping out this chapter, the first study comparing America's educational achievement to that of a later-start country (Denmark) was published by the US National Bureau of Economic Research. *The Gift of Time? School Starting Age and Mental Health* draws the conclusion that early school starting age may adversely affect educational results because there is a significantly higher incidence of attention deficit problems in children who start formal education at an early age.

ADHD, which was first identified as a 'condition' in the early 1980s, is now the second most prevalent childhood complaint in the USA (the first is asthma). The UK isn't far behind: prescriptions here for Ritalin and similar drugs have more than doubled in the last ten years. Interestingly, there isn't much of a market for Ritalin in Finland, where ADHD is comparatively rare. I'd argue that's because real play is encouraged, and children aren't expected to sit at a desk and attend to their books until they're physically, emotionally and socially mature enough to do so.

Seven-year-old children who've been allowed plenty of opportunites to play for the second half of their time on earth are far more likely to benefit from formal education than four or five year olds who, half *their* life-span ago, were still in nappies. For both lucky and unlucky children, a carefree introduction to the educational process – supported by knowledgeable, caring adults – is also likely to support the development of resilience, self-confidence and lifelong mental health.

Why we have to care about care

I hope the real experts in early years theory and practice will excuse the presumption of a literacy specialist in championing their cause. My excuse is that my admiration for skilled early years practitioners is boundless. It seems to me that the capacity to combine knowledge about child development with highly attuned attention to the children in their care is a very special talent, which should be valued by anyone who cares about the future of society. One of my aims in writing this book has been to alert as wide a readership as possible to the significance of early years experts' academic knowledge and early years practitioners' professional role in supporting young children's physical and psychological development.

Yet, despite a mountain of scientific evidence about the long-term social importance of early childhood education and care, the voice of experts in early years education is seldom heard – and even more seldom afforded public or political attention. This is particularly the case in countries with an early school starting age, where their early years expertise is considered 'relevant' for only a couple of years and their voices are increasingly drowned out by advocates of early 'schoolification'. The element of 'childcare' in early childhood education and care is therefore still regarded by most adults as little more than babysitting.

An essential quality in anyone caring for young children – and, indeed, in all the caring professions – is 'attunement', but unfortunately it's so far been very difficult to define in scientific terms. I was therefore really pleased when this word began appearing in psychological literature a few years ago, because it makes it much easier to explain what early years educators actually *do* all day. Previously, I'd relied on a term coined by the Cambridge Professor of Psychology, Simon Baron-Cohen: 'E-type thought'. 'E' is short for 'empathy', and E-type thinking is what we do when we tune in to other people's minds and see the world from their point of view.

It's relatively easy to tune in to the minds of people like ourselves – our own age-group, for example, or someone who shares our background or interests – but much more difficult with people who have very different experiences or outlook. And not many adults can tune into the minds of young children, whose mental processes are very different from those of our own. This, however, is exactly what effective early years practitioners do – it's how they know how to seize the moment and support children in ways that are appropriate for their developmental level.

Until the significance of attunement and its importance in ensuring the wellbeing of the next generation is widely recognised, I don't hold out much hope of changing political attitudes to early years education. Sadly, if Simon Baron-Cohen is right, anyone who wants to be a politician is probably trapped in another – much more ancient – paradigm. And I fear it's one from which they'll find it very difficult to escape.

The S/E dichotomy

Baron-Cohen maintains there is another broad category of human thought – the 'S-type' variety, in which 'S' stands for systemising. Every obvious aspect of human culture (such as scientific, political, economic and social systems) is based on S-type thought. Throughout history, it's been the obvious driving force of economic and cultural progress, and education systems around the world have been developed to make everyone better at it.

Not surprisingly, therefore, we tend to value S-type systemising much more highly than E-type attunement. It's probably why the Finnish educational establishment hasn't recognised the contribution of early years practice to Finland's academic success. It's also why early years experts in the UK are right at the bottom of the academic pecking order and considered slightly *infra dig* by those higher up the educational hierarchy. The E-type skills upon which successful childcare depends simply *don't fit* into an S-type paradigm.

However, the ability to empathise is just as vital for human progress as the ability to systemise. Without the human strengths it engenders – such as trust and cooperation – human beings wouldn't be able to work together and none of our clever systems would have got off the ground in the first place. Indeed, if there hadn't been well-attuned E-type thinkers (usually known as 'mothers') to care for them when they were very small, the brilliant S-typers who've driven human progress would probably have perished in infancy.

But while some man-made systems have led to progress – furthering civilisation and the spread of democracy – others have taken the human race in the other direction. Without the counter-balance of E-type thought, the S-type variety can become cold and ruthless: recent examples include the highly efficient systems devised by Hitler, Stalin and Pol Pot. So far, the human potential for both E- and S-type thought has kept the species on a generally upward track but around seventy years ago we invented the ultimate S-type thinking machine – the computer – and since then its data-generating potential has been on the exponential curve predicted by Moore's Law. As S-type thought proliferated, the E-type variety has been steadily devalued and the balance is now way out of synch. It's therefore a matter of urgency that talented S-typers start listening to what their E-type counterparts have to tell them, or we might systemise the entire species out of existence.

In terms of *Upstart*'s argument, the problem is that S-type thinkers don't have the first idea how to *care* for young children. A typical S-typer's approach to care is to produce policy documents, measurement and accountability procedures, databases and financial spreadsheets, the sort of thing that currently keeps E-type carers so busy that they don't have time to do their jobs. Systemisers are also good at inventing new products and using psychological know-how to sell them to us. And, since E-type thought has such low status, the S-typers simply can't understand why the caring professions aren't using all their magnificent data and products to raise their game.

Both types of human thought are, of course, necessary to keep the human race on an upward trajectory and isn't anybody's fault that the S/E equation has got so out of balance. I reckon it's basically a simple problem of communication. Perhaps concepts like 'attunement' and 'E-type thought' will help skilled systemisers see that they're stuck in an S-biased paradigm and find ways to winkle themselves out...

Can cultures change?

When you're trapped in a paradigm, it's very difficult to imagine any alternative. Say, for instance, a few opinion-formers in an early-start country did decide it'd be a good idea to raise the school starting age and introduce a kindergarten stage like the one in Finland. What could they do about it?

If they want to escape from an S-type mindset, one thing I'd definitely not recommend is setting up a committee to discuss all the logistical and administrative problems, including the difficulty of unpicking innumerable culturally entrenched institutional attitudes. It would probably lead to several years of discussion documents, statistical surveys, sub-committee reports and feasibility studies, until they found something else to worry about instead. Neither would I recommend an immediate in-depth economic discussion, because the chances are that, after several hours of gloomy contemplation, involving words like 'recession' and 'austerity', they'd all want to go home and pull the covers over their heads.

No, the only way to make progress would be for those opinion-formers to start by *changing their minds*. To shrug off the prejudices, fears and habits of a lifetime and, with one bound, free themselves to think the unthinkable. The first step in any culture change is to believe in the possibility of change. It's the power of belief that makes things happen, not committees or feasibility studies. After all, why *shouldn't* it be possible for an early-start country to learn from the experiences of countries like Finland and adopt as many of their good practices as immediate circumstances allow, then keep moving onwards and upwards until they too provide the best possible care and education for their youngest citizens? Since a country's children *are* that country's future, a paradigm shift of this kind is undoubtedly in everyone's long-term interests.

As a resident of Scotland, I know that sudden cultural transformation of this kind can happen. In the summer of 2014, there was a phenomenal collective 'change of mind' in my adoptive country, resulting in a level of public interest in the independence referendum that no one – even those most closely involved in Scottish politics – could previously have imagined. In the months before the vote, everyone, everywhere (from teenagers to great-grandparents) seemed to be debating the issues and discussing the future. And, many months later, that optimistic spirit of democractic engagement still seems to be abroad in the land.

It certainly inspired me to crack on with the book. And as soon as *Upstart's* finished, I hope to be working full-time with like-minded parents and professionals to launch an '*Upstart Scotland*' campaign. We believe we can convince our countrymen and women to lead the way in early years education and make Scotland the first UK nation to create 'a good society' by doing the best for its little children.

Why culture shift needs legal aid

I know one of the first questions *Upstart Scotland* will be asked is why transforming early years practice requires a change in the law. Why can't we just change the emphasis of education for the under-sevens? Indeed, the Scottish *Curriculum for Excellence* covers the years three to eighteen, and takes a developmental approach to education which is considerably less prescriptive than the English National Curriculum. Many figures in the educational establishment will doubtless claim that 'we're doing it already' – but we're not. If we were, small Scottish children would not be struggling to read, write and do sums before they're developmentally competent. There must, of course, be a point at which such 'schooling' begins – and I hope *Upstart* has satisfactorily explained why that should be set at seven.

The recent experience of another Celtic nation demonstrates how deeply the top-down philosophy is entrenched in UK educational culture. Until 1997, the education system in Wales was broadly similar to England's but after the devolution of powers to the Welsh Assembly its first education minister (Jane Davidson) was prepared to listen to early years experts. For a while, it seemed that Wales might break away from Britain's traditionally early start on formal learning. They abandoned SAT tests for seven year olds and began introducing a Foundation Phase for children aged three to seven, to be based on a developmental model.

However, the Welsh early years sector soon found itself going through the same 'blood and feathers' process as their English counterparts (see Chapter 1). Practitioners piloting the project from 2001 struggled to reconcile their 'bottom-up' developmental approach with 'top-down' demands from the primary sector, which was still required to follow the National Curriculum. So when the Foundation Phase was rolled out nationally in 2008, the accompanying document was distinctly schizophrenic. It began with the claim that 'at the centre of the statutory curriculum framework lies the holistic development of children', but finished with comprehensive lists of expected 'outcomes', including a great many specific literacy and numeracy skills.

It doesn't matter whether practitioners working with the under-sevens are required to aim at 'targets', 'goals' or 'outcomes'. Any requirement to focus on highly specific skills by a particular age is at odds with the principles of 'holistic development'. To revisit the argument introduced in Chapter 1: kindergarten education and formal schooling are fundamentally different. The former is based on a child-centred model; the latter inevitably moves toward a more curriculum-centred approach. Bottom-up versus top-down. Kindergarten practitioners develop individual children's all-round potential as learners and human beings; school teachers teach specific skills and knowledge to specific age-groups of pupils.

By 2010, the dream of a genuinely developmentally appropriate Welsh Foundation Stage was knocked on the head by the introduction of a National Framework for Literacy and Numeracy, with targets for five year olds, followed by standardised tests at seven that I reckon are even more demanding than the English SATs. Five years later, the Welsh government launched yet *another* review of education based on yet another report – *Successful Futures*. This noted support for the idea of a Foundation Stage but also recommended 'Achievement Outcomes' beginning at age five.

The lesson is that, if kindergarten is to have the beneficial effects it currently delivers in Finland, Estonia and Switzerland, the years between three and seven must be – *and be seen to be* – a completely separate stage in children's education. To achieve a genuine paradigm shift, a nation's electorate must require its government to make the grandest (and among the cheapest) of political gestures: a change in the law.

In fact, there's plenty of evidence that, in modern democracies, any significant change in cultural attitudes – such as public responses to drink-driving, corporal punishment, gender equality, smoking and so on – require legislative support. A change in the law signals a change in the national value-system. It raises awareness of the issues. And it ensures that *everyone* engages with the paradigm shift.

What about the bottom line?

If the law is changed, there are clearly economic implications. We'd have to ensure:

- funding for three to four years of kindergarten education for all children
- appropriate buildings and facilities for the care and education of children aged three to seven, including regular access to outdoor play space
- a workforce with the professional knowledge and personal skills to support children's development.

With luck, that wouldn't be too difficult to get under way.

- There's already an established budget for the education of four, five and six year olds in the UK and money has already been earmarked to subsidise part-time nursery education for three year olds (in the first couple of years, research suggests that part-time attendance at kindergarten is in fact preferable to a full day away from a home environment).

- Existing facilities, including nurseries and the early years departments of primary schools, can be adapted for use as kindergartens and gradually improved, and increased access to outdoor play space could involve imaginative use of local parks, playgrounds, wild places and other community resources.

- There's also already an established early years workforce and, although further training is clearly necessary (especially support for primary-trained teachers of five- and six-year-olds in moving from a 'top-down' transmission model of education to a 'bottom-up' developmental model), this could be provided in the initial stages via in-service courses. These could include 'distance learning' resources, with video illustration and internet-based discussion. Specific kindergarten teaching qualifications could be phased in over time.

It seems to me that the bottom line in the immediate future relates to ethos, rather than economics. Kindergarten education is play-based and developmentally appropriate – a bottom-up, child-centred ethos, as opposed to the more curriculum-centred ethos of school. In making that 'ethical' change, the government and educational establishment will be sending out a strong message to parents and the general public about the developmental needs of young children, especially the need for play (including regular outdoor play).

There's no lack of expertise to draw on – the UK already has a long tradition of excellent early years practice, inspired by pioneers such as Margaret McMillan and Susan Isaacs, and in Scotland there's been a long-standing commitment to the Froebelian approach. As public understanding about the importance of early childhood grows, it will be possible to extend other support to families of young children, as in Finland. And remember, Finland's system wasn't built in a day – it's taken forty years to achieve the current state of play. Costs can be spread over the long term, as the kindergarten system is gradually improved – hopefully, as time goes on, with more purpose-built facilities.

Since arithmetic is not my forte, I have to leave the fine detail of financing these measures to accomplished number-crunchers. But even a non-mathematician like me can see that any initial investment would soon be off-set by savings in terms of spending on special educational needs and the cost of dealing with children's mental and physical health problems. And that, in the long-term, providing what the under-sevens *really* need should lead to massive savings in the budgets for education, health, social services and criminal justice.

Politics isn't my forte either, so sorting out all the pride, prejudice and vested interests of 150 years, and ensuring that the new system can work must also be someone else's problem. However that should be much easier if ethics, rather than economics, is recognised as the bottom line. What's at stake here is the next generation's health and wellbeing, the potential for all children – whatever their background – to succeed at school and an opportunity to build a 'good society'. If those ethical principles can be kept before the politicians, union officials, educationists, CEOs of NGOs, civil servants and all other members of committees and sub-committees, perhaps they'll be motivated to get on with it.

It's not just the economy, stupid

Economic considerations can't be ignored, but as long as we always think of 'the bottom line' in purely financial terms, there's no chance of making what politicians these days call 'transformational change'. Most of the problems confronting children, society – and, indeed, our world – are due to the relentless focus on economic growth over the last three or four decades. Researching and writing about small children has made me very aware that, as argued in Chapters 3 and 5, the most important things in life cannot be bought in the shops – which is why 'love' and 'play' are four-letter words in economic circles. And as developmental psychologist Sue Gerhart argues in her book *The Selfish Society: How we forgot to love one another and made money instead* it's the way we *care* for young children (and their society) that determines whether they thrive. 'Care', of course, is another four-letter word.

In twenty-first-century western societies, early childcare is increasingly provided outside the home. Given mounting neuroscientific evidence about the significance of the pre-school years, ethical considerations about the quality of childcare *must* count at least as much as economic ones. And, since care and education are intricately entwined, the educational ethos of institutions catering for three- to seven-year olds is supremely important. So, while I hope *Upstart* has produced strong economic *and* educational arguments for raising the school starting age and providing what the under-sevens *really* need, these pale in comparison with the ethical ones. Young children's wellbeing should always trump financial considerations and holistic education (for lifelong learning) trumps the pursuit of 'school readiness'.

At the moment, we're trapped in the middle of a paradigmatic Venn diagram:

- The early-start paradigm means that our under-sevens get one or two years of (often inadequate) nursery education and two years of inappropriately formal schooling, rather than the three/four years of the developmentally appropriate kindergarten education they need.
- The S-type thought paradigm (almost certainly encouraged by too-early schooling) means our politicians keep tinkering with the early-start system, accumulating data about it and devising extra systems to solve problems, rather than

recognising that the whole thing is fundamentally flawed and needs restructuring by people who actually understand how young children think and learn (since that involves E-type thought, it is, of course, unthinkable in S-type terms).

- The It's-The-Economy paradigm means that all discussion of the resultant problems is framed within a monetary context: children and staff are seen as 'human capital'; progress and success are measured in terms of accounts and accountability; the only thing that matters as much as money is data.

Meanwhile, the data informs us that the achievement gap is widening, mental health problems among children and young people are spiralling out of control and our educational results are nowhere near as impressive as those of countries with play-based kindergartens. Neither are our records on tackling crime, relationship breakdown, gender discrimination or social justice in general.

We are a society profoundly out of balance, obsessed with systems, statistics and monetary measures of success. It's meant we've steadily lost faith in the human strengths (kindness, trust, cooperation) that underpin social health and wellbeing. But we could escape from our triple-paradigm trap by prioritising kindness in our treatment of little children, allowing them a few carefree years of play before they start school. And we could reaffirm faith in human nature by trusting their ability to learn from play – especially when supported by a highly attuned and well-qualified early years workforce. In fact, if enough adults were to work together to achieve this particular cultural shift, their collective change of mind would immediately make us a more balanced (and, eventually, even a 'good') society. In the words of Nelson Mandela, 'there can be no keener revelation of a society's soul than the way in which it treats its children.'

***

There's no doubt the twenty-first century will be challenging, so today's adults have the grave responsibility of raising a generation that can face those challenges bravely and work together to overcome them, whatever they may be. Like every generation before them, they'll need to be adaptable, resilient, accomplished problem-solvers, with the patience to pursue long-term ends rather than immediate rewards. They'll need to be confident learners, skilled communicators, able to cooperate and collaborate but also to think for themselves.

When a small child is making weird mixtures in a mud kitchen or designing 'dinosaur traps', it may seem to have little connection with the capacity to survive and thrive in an uncertain future. When they're singing nursery rhymes in a kindergarten circle, snuggling up to listen to a story or counting trees on a visit to the woods it may seem irrelevant to their future educational success. But this is how nature – including human nature – designed children to learn.

The first seven years are for play, not school. With time and space to play, children grow up bright, balanced, ready to live and learn with joy and hope. Without it, the future will look increasingly bleak.

For children's sake, and for sake of all our futures, thank you for reading *Upstart* – and please start helping to make the change *NOW!*

Appendices

APPENDIX 1:

School starting ages around the world

On the facing page is a table listing countries like the United Kingdom where children start school at age five, and countries where they start at age seven. In all other unlisted countries, children start school at age six.

(**C**) indicates a member of the Commonwealth. These countries have an historical relationship to the United Kingdom.

Source: The World Bank –
http://data.worldbank.org/indicator/SE.PRM.AGES

Age 5	Age 7
Antigua and Barbuda (**C**)	Afghanistan
Australia (**C**)	Brazil
The Bahamas (**C**)	Bulgaria
Belize (**C**)	Burundi
Cayman Islands (**C**)	China
Dominica (**C**)	Croatia
Grenada (**C**)	El Salvador
Ireland	Equatorial Guinea
Malta (**C**)	Eritrea
Mauritius (**C**)	Estonia
Myanmar (formerly Burma)	Finland
Nepal	The Gambia
New Zealand (**C**)	Guatemala
Pakistan (**C**)	Guinea
Samoa (**C**)	Hungary
Sri Lanka (**C**)	Indonesia
St Kitts and Nevis (**C**)	Kazakhstan
Saint Lucia (**C**)	Korea Dem. Republic
St Vincent and the Grenadines (**C**)	Kyrgyz Republic
Tonga (**C**)	Latvia
Trinidad and Tobago (**C**)	Liechtenstein
United Kingdom (**C**)	Lithuania
	Mali
	Namibia (**C**)
	Niger
	Papua New Guinea (**C**)
	Poland
	Romania
	Russian Federation
	Rwanda (**C**)
	Senegal
	Serbia
	South Africa (**C**)
	Sweden
	Switzerland
	Tajikistan
	Tanzania (**C**)
	Turkmenistan
	Uzbekistan
	Zambia (**C**)

Appendix 2:
Early education in early-start nations

Scotland

The school starting age is five but Scottish children are slightly older when they enter P1 (Primary 1) than English children entering the reception class (Year R) (see Appendix 5 for details). Pre-school education in Scotland is, as throughout the UK, a mixture of state and private provision, all subject to centralised regulation. There is not, however, anything resembling the Early Years Foundation Stage (*EYFS*) because Scotland's *Curriculum for Excellence* (*CfE*) covers children's education between the ages of three and eighteen.

Like its many accompanying policy documents, *CfE* is based on a developmental progression which acknowledges an Early Years stage (up to age eight as in United Nations documentation). However, in practice, formal schooling in Scotland generally begins in P1, for the same historical and cultural reasons as in England.

Until recently, school-based assessment was not officially related to children's age but the adoption of age-related targets has meant this has seldom been the case. Some local authorities already use standardised baseline tests when children start school and in 2015 the Scottish government announced that national tests in literacy would be introduced, starting at age five.

Wales

Before 1997, the education system in Wales was similar to that of England (with the addition of Welsh language teaching, starting in some schools at five). However, after devolution of powers to the Welsh Assembly, their approach to education became more individual, and included abandonment of the Key Stage 1 tests and the introduction of a Foundation Phase for three to seven –year olds, intended to be based on the Nordic model.

My impressions of the Foundation Phase's progress are given in Chapter 7 (Why culture shift needs legal aid). In brief, it was a brave initiative but in the long run doesn't appear to have helped Wales escape the schoolification process. Literacy and numeracy tests for seven year olds were reintroduced after a poor Programme for International Student Assessment (PISA) result in 2010.

Northern Ireland

With a starting age of four, Northern Ireland has always sent its children to school earlier than anywhere in the world. However, the first two years (P1 and P2) are designated the Foundation Stage and the NI National Curriculum states that children of this age should 'experience most of their education through well-supported and challenging play'.

The programme of study for children in the Foundation Stage was influenced by European practice (via NI's 'Enriched Curriculum' project around the turn of the century) and is less demanding in terms of expected outcomes than the *EYFS*. There may be a connection between this and NI's better performance in international surveys of educational achievement than other UK countries. However, others would argue that NI's success is due to retention of the 11plus and selective secondary education.

Australia

Until recently, educational provision was the responsibility of the individual states of Australia and there was considerable variation. At present however, a National Curriculum is being phased in, covering the years five to eighteen. As in the UK, there has been considerable expansion of pre-school facilities in recent decades, provided by both the state and private companies.

By law, Australian children must be enrolled in school by their sixth birthday, with most arriving not long after they're five but the actual starting age varies from state to state. In 2015, there was a suggestion in the state of Tasmania that the school starting age should be lowered to four, which was fiercely opposed by Early Childhood Australia.

The first year at school, which used to be known as 'kindergarten' in some states, is now to be universally described as the Foundation Year. Detailed lists of Achievement Standards for the National Curriculum include expectations of children's performance in the Foundation

Year which are similar to those for UK five year olds. As a long-time admirer of Western Australia's First Steps programme, which is based on developmental principles, I suspect a much more formal approach will now be necessary to ensure most Foundation pupils reach the new Achievement Standards.

So far, Australia has been the highest performing of the early-start countries in PISA surveys and the only one in which the achievement gap has not widened. It will be interesting to note whether this situation changes in the light of creeping schoolification.

New Zealand

Education in New Zealand isn't compulsory until children are six, although most start school when they turn five. Before that, there is an Early Years Curriculum, 'Te Whāriki', which has been in place since 1996 for settings covering the care of children from birth to school entry. This was designed as a 'holistic, integrated' curriculum and settings were not required to aim for particular learning outcomes. In recent years, however, there has been increased emphasis on assessment.

Once in school, children follow a National Curriculum, first introduced in the early 1990s. The first two years (for five and six year olds) are grouped together as Curriculum Level 1, with achievement objectives for the three Rs similar to those in the UK and Australia. As in other early-start countries, parental anxiety about these objectives leads to pressure for children to read and write at an increasingly early age.

While the general pattern of early schooling seems similar to England, there is one interesting divergence: some Steiner-Waldorf schools in NZ (which don't start formal teaching until children are seven) are state-funded so it's currently possible for children from a variety of economic backgrounds to have four years of play-based kindergarten education.

USA

There is considerable variation in educational policy and practice between states in the USA. Nationally, however, the school starting age is six, although five-year-old children are entitled to a year in Grade K, which stands for kindergarten. This is taken up by the overwhelming majority of children.

Until the turn of the century, most US kindergarten provision was similar to European approach described in Chapter 1, but this has changed due to current policy. The 'Common Core curriculum', introduced in 2010, covers K-12 and includes standards for literature and maths, similar to those in the *EYFS*. By 2014 its principles had been adopted by 43 states.

In recent years, the US government has also offered pre-K education for four year olds but funding is available only for selected providers. The 'schoolification' resulting from Common Core now affects pre-K classes (for children of four and under), which are subsidised for children from disadvantaged homes. This makes it increasingly difficult for practitioners to follow practice guidelines such as those issued by the National Association for the Education of Young Children.

Appendix 3:
The UK Early Childhood Forum's Charter

The Early Childhood Forum is an alliance of (currently) 34 organisations, including professional bodies such as Early Education, the National Association of Headteachers, the Association of Educational Psychologists and large third sector organisations, such as the National Children's Bureau.

I'm including its 2014 Charter for Early Childhood here to illustrate the widespread concern about early childhood policy in the UK among professionals in the sector, including their consensus that the 'early years phase' should extend to age seven (see points 7 and 10–12).

ECF Charter for Early Childhood

The Early Childhood Forum (ECF) brings together membership organisations from across the early childhood sector to debate issues, celebrate differences and develop consensus. Together, we champion all young children and their families, promote inclusion and challenge inequalities, discrimination and prejudice.

Our 12-point charter aims to influence the manifestos of all the political parties. Several member organisations have produced their own manifestos and we encourage the whole sector to seek areas for consensus to guide politicians in their decision-making, using the latest evidence from research and practice.

1. Agreement to set up an all-party planning and funding group to develop and implement long-term policy for young children's education, health and care.

2. A demonstrated commitment to multi-professional working across education, health and care based on evidence and informed by research and professional guidance from practitioners.
3. Consistent, well-funded and effective policies that give parents and carers real choices about whether to stay at home.
4. Universal access to children's centres and related services as a vital route to family support programmes and outreach for vulnerable families or those in crisis.
5. Support for family and child physical and mental health through equitable universal implementation of the health programmes.
6. Formative assessment throughout early childhood to support families and professionals to provide the best possible care and education.
7. A statutory framework for early years from birth extended to age seven that is coherent and appropriately developed and elaborated for different stages within it.
8. Guidance that acknowledges each child's unique requirements at every stage of development and that recognises the importance of consistent loving care from a main carer in a nurturing environment.
9. A presumption for fully funded inclusion for disabled children and those with special educational needs. Early years providers must have access to specialist support and qualified Special Educational Needs Coordinators (SENCOs), as in schools.
10. A commitment to work towards universal high-quality integrated education, health and care whilst strengthening the entitlement for children in early years to access play and daily outdoor experiences in all provision until age seven.
11. A specialist qualification route which includes graduate staff who are qualified to work in the early years phase (birth to age seven) with a clearly defined pay and career structure and a statutory requirement to participate in continuous professional development.
12. Integrated inspections that are carried out by qualified and knowledgeable inspectors, who have had experience of working with children under age seven.

Beliefs and principles

ECF believes that early childhood is a crucial stage of life and that:

- the needs of the infant and child must be placed at the centre of the planning and provision of high-quality services.

- all children are entitled to participation, provision, play and protection, as outlined in the UN Convention on the Rights of the Child and to live without fear of discrimination.
- the safety and wellbeing of children is central to every aspect of children's learning, health and development.
- knowledge and understanding of child development is fundamental for all practitioners who work with young children.
- parents and the home environment have the strongest influence on children's development.
- learning is a process of development through interaction and experience that begins before birth.
- young children should have equal rights to culturally and developmentally appropriate play-based provision, both indoors and outdoors, that develops their understanding, dispositions, skills and knowledge.
- every child needs sensitive, attuned and responsive care in the first years of life and a key person to support them.
- all parents need support at times to feel confident in raising their children in a loving and supportive environment.

ECF promotes the principle that a child's best interests are paramount (Children Act 1989) and children have human rights to family life, privacy and dignity (Human Rights Act 1998).

Elements in current policy and practice work against this principle and are barriers to enabling early years practitioners to focus on their key role. For example, the focus on summative assessment, testing and league tables takes staff away from time spent developing relationships with children.

Investing in early years is critical. National and international evidence shows the cost benefits to the public purse of investing in early years for longer-term social and economic gains. Fair, devolved funding per child in their early years is needed to improve the health, wellbeing and educational experiences for all children.

Appendix 4:
The phonemes of English

The table overleaf shows the phonemes of English as defined by the UK National Literacy Strategy in the Progression in Phonics training materials. It gives a sense of their complexity.

Consonant phonemes with consistent spellings	Consonant phonemes with alternative spellings
/b/ **b**at, ra**bb**it /d/ **d**og, da**dd**y /g/ **g**irl, gi**gg**le /h/ **h**ot /l/ **l**og, lo**ll**y /m/ **m**at, su**mm**er /n/ **n**ut, di**nn**er /p/ **p**ig, su**pp**er /r/ **r**at, ca**rr**y /t/ **t**op, pa**tt**er /y/ **y**ellow /th/ **th**is (voiced) **th**ing (unvoiced)	/k/ **c**at, **k**ing, ba**ck**, s**ch**ool, **q**ueen (also the /k/ sound in bo**x**) /s/ **s**un, pre**ss**, **c**ircle (also /s/ in bo**x**) /f/ **f**un, **ph**oto /j/ **j**am, **g**inger, bri**dge** /w/ **w**orm, q**u**een /z/ **z**oo, pin**s**, **x**ylophone /v/ **v**an (one exception: o**f**) /sh/ **sh**eep, sta**ti**on, **ch**ef /ch/ **ch**in, it**ch** /ng/ si**ng**, pi**n**k /zh/ mea**s**ure, a**z**ure

'Short' and 'long' vowel phonemes	Other vowel phonemes
/a/ b**a**g /e/ b**e**t, br**ea**d, s**ai**d /i/ b**i**g, c**y**linder /o/ t**o**p, w**a**s /u/ b**u**n, l**o**ve /ae/ d**ay**, p**ai**n, g**a**te, gr**ea**t /ee/ f**ee**t, s**ea**t, P**e**te, m**e** /ie/ t**ie**, t**igh**t, fl**y**, t**i**me /oa/ b**oa**t, gr**ow**, b**o**ne, t**oe**, g**o** /ue/ bl**ue**, m**oo**n, gr**ew**, fl**u**te, y**ou**	/oo/ g**oo**d, p**u**t, c**ou**ld, w**o**lf ur/ch**ur**ch, b**ir**d, h**er**b, **ear**th, w**or**d /ar/ st**ar**t, f**a**ther /or/ c**or**n, d**oor**, sh**ore**, r**oar**, y**our** /aw/ p**aw**, t**au**t, t**a**ll, t**a**lk, t**augh**t /ow/ cl**ow**n, sh**ou**t /oy/ b**oy**, **oi**l /ear/ n**ear**, d**eer**, h**ere** /air/ ch**air**, sh**are**, th**ere** 'schwa', as in farm**er**, doct**or**, gramm**ar**, met**re**, col**our**, Americ**a**...

Appendix 5:
Summerborns and winterborns

Admission dates in UK countries

In England and Wales, where children are required to start school in the September before they turn five, children born on August 31 are expected to be enrolled in the reception class the day after their fourth birthday. Parents of 'summerborn' children can apply to defer entry, but this is at the discretion of the local authority. Usually, if children do defer entry they miss the reception year and go straight into Year 1.

In Northern Ireland, children who are four before July 1 begin school that September, so those with July and August birthdays are almost five when they enter P1. On the other hand, a child born on June 30 is only just four.

In Scotland the youngest in a class are 'winterborns' because children born between March and August start school in the August following their fifth birthday. Most children born between September and February follow the same rule, but it's possible for parents of winterborns to defer entry until the following year. Deferment is automatically granted for children born in January and February, but is otherwise at the discretion of the local authority, some of which are more amenable than others.

The 'youngest in the class' dilemma

There is evidence that, on the whole, younger children *everywhere* fare less well throughout their school careers than their older classmates, whatever the school starting age. Bigger, more mature, more confident children just have a natural advantage over the rest of their year group. However, the older children are when they start school, the less significant this natural disadvantage is.

The 'youngest in the class' dilemma is, for obvious reasons, a particular problem in early-start nations – and a serious one, because it's now been shown that these children are much more likely to be identified as having special educational needs and/or mental health problems as time goes on. However, local authorities are often reluctant to defer school entry because of funding issues (children are entitled to a certain number of years in education and, if they start school a year late, the local authority has to fund an extra year of pre-school education). This is why many English local authorities insist that 'deferred children' should go straight into the Y1 class. Since this means they miss a full year of primary education, deferment can also put summerborns at a disadvantage.

Add to this the potential social and emotional problems for children who are separated from their friends when parents 'hold them back' for a further year in pre-school. One way or another, it seems that in early-start countries the date of a child's birth may have serious long-term repercussions whatever action parents take.

Recent developments

In recent years, evidence about the long-term disadvantages for summerborns has become increasingly available. Parents campaigning for deferral in England and Northern Ireland (see www.summerbornchildren.org in England and www.parentsoutloud.com for NI) have therefore become increasingly vocal.

In December 2014, after consultations with parents and union representatives, the Northern Ireland government announced plans to increase flexibility about school starting ages. It then unaccountably dropped the plans in April 2015, meaning that parental concern in NI is likely to grow.

In England, in September 2015, the Schools Minister also announced that local authorities should revise their policy on deferment, making it easier for parents to hold their child back a year. As yet, there has been no retraction so it remains to be seen whether (and how) the policies will be put into practice in 2016.

The Welsh school admission policy is separate from England's and as yet there has been no indication as to whether Wales will follow the English government's lead. Information about deferment in Wales is available on www.bliss.org.uk.

In Scotland, where the starting date means children are not quite so young on school entry and many local authorities are flexible about deferment, parental anxiety has so far been less widespread.

However, informed parents are increasingly opting to defer school entry and there have been battles with less flexible local authorities (see www.takingparentsseriously.wordpress.com).

USA

In the USA, parents are entitled to defer their children's entry to the kindergarten class (see Appendix 2), a practice known as 'red-shirting'. As kindergarten has become increasingly schoolified, an increasing number of parents have taken advantage of this entitlement and a 2015 study (The Gift of Time? – see Chapter 7, The paradigm trap) suggested that around a fifth of children are now 'red-shirts', meaning that they start kindergarten at age six, rather than five.

As most of these parents appear to be well-educated and middle-class, some commentators have suggested that this is connected with the publication of Malcolm Gladwell's book *The Outliers,* in which he claims that the oldest children in a class tend to be higher achievers in practically every field (i.e. it is an aspect of 'pushy parenting'). Others claim that parents simply don't believe their children are socially and emotionally ready to start formal schooling.

Appendix 6:
A Finnish kindergarten's lesson for linguistic skills

This briefing paper for visitors was supplied by the teacher of a pre-primary class (six-year-olds) – see page 147 for a description of the actual lesson. The brevity and flexibility of her 'Lesson Objectives' show how, rather than spending hours in meticulous planning and other accountability procedures, she is trusted to exercise professional judgement in providing the most appropriate support for each individual child. Finland's consistently high scores in international surveys indicate that, with this age-group, a developmentally appropriate approach leads to better long-term outcomes than the top-down, curriculum-focussed teaching to which five and six year olds are subjected in early-start countries.

Helsinki, 6 May 2015

Background information

The children in the group are at different reading stages. Some of the children read fluently, some can read short syllables and a few are still practising recognising letters. The lesson is planned in a way that takes into account all of the different stages of reading the children are currently in. We particularly want to encourage feelings of accomplishment and learning.

Throughout the entire year we have practised recognising different feelings and how to talk openly about them. In this lesson we want to address the feeling of *nervousness* especially because it is a very current topic amongst the children (starting school, acquiring new friends, etc.).

These matters will be processed through *play and movement*.

Lesson objectives

- Letter, syllable, word, sentence: taking into account every child's stage of reading development
- Discussing a certain feeling.

Structure of the lesson (may change direction according to the children's responses)

- Recognising *current feeling*, telling about it
- Discussion about *feeling nervous*
- Setting *play* in motion
- *Sportive play* with letters, syllables, words and sentences

NOTES AND REFERENCES

Books in print (referenced by author's name) are listed in the Bibliography

CHAPTER ONE

A very British story
• Worldwide school starting ages – data.worldbank.org/indicator/SE.PRM.AGES
• English starting age – Caroline Sharp, *School Starting Age: European policy and recent research*, NFER (2002) www.nfer.ac.uk/nfer/publications/44410/44410.pdf
• Victorian politicians – Royal Commission on the State of Popular Education in England, Parliamentary Papers (1861)
    —Derek Gillard, *Education in England: a brief history* (2011) www.educationengland.org.uk/history
• Twentieth-century educational developments – the 'standards' controversy is outlined in more detail in 'The Primary Wars', Chapter 1 (page 15)
• 'Bums on seats' – Sue Palmer, 'Reclaiming Reception', *Child Education* (2005)

Everyone out of step but us
• Hugh Cunningham quote – Cunningham (2006)
• 'The first seven years are for play' – I was first told about the prophet Mohammed's advice at a Moslem conference in 2006, where I had been invited to speak about *Toxic Childhood*. Since then, many Moslem friends have reiterated it, usually in the form of words I give in this chapter
    —See www.sajedeen.org/resources/sisters-section/157-bringing-up-children-aged-1-to-7-according-to-principles-of-islam
• 'Japanese aphorism' – when I mentioned Mohammed's quote at a conference in Japan in 2007, several people came to tell me about this one. I've been told that many other peoples around the world have similar sayings, including Native Americans and Australians, but haven't been able to find written references. The famous Jesuit quotation is referenced in Chapter 2 (page 45)
    — See also www.ceser.hyogo-u.ac.jp/suzukimj/paper9_99/paper9_99.html
• European educationists – Elkind (2015)
• Piaget and Vygotsky – for a summary of the similarities and differences between these two developmental psychologists, including their agreement that seven is a

critical age in terms of educational provision, see psychology.wikia.com/wiki/
Similarities_%26_differences_between_Piaget_%26_Vygotsky_theories

The power of play

• An overview of recent science about play –The National Institute for Play (USA)
www.nifplay.org/science/pattern-play/
    —Also websites of the various UK Play Associations www.playengland.org.uk;
www.playscotland.org; www.playwales.org.uk; www.playboard.org (NI)
• Play and early education –Whitebread (2012), Brock et al (2014)
• The significance of play in early learning – see Chapter 2

The quest for the three Rs

• Matthew Arnold quote – Alexander (2001)
• Education during the twentieth century – Paul Bolton, *House of Commons
Educational Statistics*, SN/SG/4252 (2012)
• Literacy and social mobility comparisons – baby boomers versus today
    www.independent.co.uk/student/news/british-education-ines-crisis-literacy-and-
numeracy-skills-of-young-people-in-uk-among-lowest-in-developed-world-8866117.html
    — See also www.theguardian.com/news/datablog/2012/may/22/social-mobility-
data-charts

The primary wars

• This section is based on my own experiences, as one who lived through these 'wars'.
In 1990, I organised a national campaign for *Balance in the Teaching of Language and
Literacy Skills* and reported on developments frequently in the educational press
during the 1990s, for example,
    — 'Let battle commence...' *Times Educational Supplement* (10 November 1995)
    — 'Between the lines' *Times Educational Supplement* (17 December 1999)

No child left behind

• Information on US policy – see the US Department of Education website www2.
ed.gov/nclb/landing.jhtml
• Birth to three framework –webarchive.nationalarchives.gov.uk/20130401151715/
http://www.education.gov.uk/publications/eOrderingDownload/BIRTHCD-PDF1.pdf
• Foundation Stage Guidance – www.qca.org.uk/160.html

More haste, more problems

• 'The Longevity Project' – Friedman (2012) www.ncbi.nlm.nih.gov/pmc/articles/
PMC2713445/ - R33
• Howard Friedman quote – from personal letter to Dr Richard House of the *Too
Much Too Soon* campaign
• Finnish/UK comparison – drawn from PISA surveys of educational achievement
since 2004 and
    —UNICEF surveys of childhood wellbeing since 2007
    —World Bank's GINI index of income equality
    —OECD's survey of family breakdown in 2012
    —'UK high on family breakdown table' *BBC News* (29 December 2012)
www.bbc.co.uk/news/uk-20863917

Why, oh why?
• Ball, *Start Right: The importance of early learning* (1995) eric.ed.gov/?id=ED372833
• *Too Much Too Soon* campaign – www.toomuchtoosoon.org
• Robin Alexander, et al., *Cambridge Primary Review* – cprtrust.org.uk/

Anglo-Saxon attitudes
• *Every Child Matters*, HMSO (2003) www.education.gov.uk/consultations/downloadableDocs/EveryChildMatters.pdf
• BBC report on highly effective nursery schools – coverage of the EPPE report (November 2004) www.ioe.ac.uk/RB_Final_Report_3-7.pdf
• First *Early Years Foundation Stage* statutory framework produced in 2008 – a short film can be found here www.youtube.com/watch?v=nmheYO0Z72o
    —The most recent edition (2014) can be found at www.foundationyears.org.uk/eyfs-statutory-framework/

CHAPTER TWO

The information in this chapter is drawn from many sources in developmental psychology, educational theory, early years practice and playwork. Specific authorities are cited in the notes below but the chapter is necessarily a digest of all I've learned in the last fifteen years.
• Intrinsic and extrinsic motivation – a useful summary in 'About Education' psychology.about.com/od/motivation/f/difference-between-extrinsic-and-intrinsic-motivation.htm

Born to learn
• Birth to three quote from top American psychologists (page 28) – Gopnik, et al. (1999)
• Three to seven – Pellis and Pellis (2010), Whitebread (2012), Brock, et al. (2014)
    —Whitebread, *The Importance of Play* (2012) www.importanceofplay.eu/IMG/pdf/dr_david_whitebread_-_the_importance_of_play.pdf
• Love and play – Over the years, I've come to the conclusion that these are the two most essential elements for childhood wellbeing. The love of adults not only keeps children safe, fed, clothed and sheltered but also provides the social and emotional support young infants need to thrive. The drive to play, coming from within the child, is the main means by which each generation moves from dependence on adult care to independent thought and action.

Birth to three – tuning in to people
• For a more detailed account of early language development – Sue Palmer, Chapter 4: It's Good To Talk, *Toxic Childhood* (2015); also Boyce (2009)
• 'Mind-mindedness'– one of various terms used by psychologists, neuroscientists and philosophers, including 'theory of mind' and, more loosely, 'empathy'. I've chosen 'mind-mindedness' because it is the term used by Elizabeth Meins and Charles Ferneyhough, whose work at Durham University on parental mind-mindedness I've followed with interest for the last decade. It links to the word 'attunement' (see next section), which seems to me an essential quality for anyone caring for young children.
• Professor Peter Hobson quote – Hobson (2002)

Birth to three – tuning in to play
• Connections between physical, social and emotional development – Goddard Blyth (2005)
• 'Play is the work of the child' – attributed to many, but Montessori is the most frequently cited authority.
• 'Well-attuned adults skilled at mind-mindedness' – C. Ferneyhough and E. Meins, et al., 'Mind-Mindedness and Theory of Mind: Mediating Roles of Language and Perspectival Symbolic Play', *Child Development* 84 (2013)

Now we are three
• Evidence that kindergarten is beneficial – E. Melhuish and K. Sylva et al., *Effective Pre-School and Primary Education, 3–11 project,* Institute of Education, University of London (2008)
   —Kathy Sylva was later quoted as saying that there is no problem in putting children of three and over into full-time nursery care, but between two and three the research is 'mixed' and below the age of two there are 'some serious and valid concerns' in Amelia Gentleman, 'The Great Nursery Debate', *Guardian* (2 October 2010)

The state of play
• UNCRC – see www.unicef.org/crc/
• Playworkers definition of play – drawn from the work of Bob Hughes and Frank King in *Best Play* (2000) www.playengland.org.uk/media/202623/best-play.pdf
   —It continues: 'Play can be fun or serious. Through play children explore social, material and imaginary worlds and their relationship with them, elaborating all the while a flexible range of responses to the challenges they encounter. By playing, children learn and develop as individuals, and as members of the community'.
• Self-regulation – shorthand for what the National Scientific Council on the Developing Child describes as the gradual maturation of the brain until 'by age seven, some of the capabilities and brain circuits underlying executive function are remarkably similar to those found in adults'.
   —From *Building the Brain's 'Air Traffic Control' System: how early experiences shape the development of executive function*, Harvard University (2011) developingchild. harvard.edu/wp-content/uploads/2011/05/How-Early-Experiences-Shape-the-Development-of-Executive-Function.pdf
• A critical element in the development of self-regulation skills – M. Hyson, C. Copple and J. Jones, 'Early childhood development and education', *Handbook of Child Psychology: Vol. 4 Child psychology in practice*, eds. K. A. Renninger and I. Sigel, Wiley (2006) www.researchconnections.org/files/childcare/pdf/PlayandApproachestoLearning-MarilouHyson-1.pdf
   —Ponitz et al., 'A Structured Observation of Behavioral Self-Regulation and its Contribution to Kindergarten Outcomes', *Developmental Psychology* (2009) people.oregonstate.edu/~mcclellm/ms/Ponitz_McClelland_Matthews_Morrison_DP09.pdf
   —David Whitebread, 'Play, Metacognition and Self-Regulation', *Play and Learning in Early Years Settings: From research to practice*, eds. J. Broadhead et al., Sage (2010)
• David Whitebread quote – Whitebread (2012)

The play's the thing
• Active play – The huge importance of active play for all aspects of development is explained in an NHS video. In it, a primary headteacher claims that play is 'essential'

until the age of five – a Finnish or Swiss headteacher would presumably claim play is 'essential' until the age of seven. Assumptions about when the play has to stop are often determined by a nation's school starting age. www.nhs.uk/video/pages/activeplay.aspx
• Pretend play – S.B. Kaufmann, 'The Need for Pretend Play in Child Development' *Psychology Today* (2015) www.psychologytoday.com/blog/beautiful-minds/201203/the-need-pretend-play-in-child-development

Team play
• Social play – Frost and Wortham, 'Summary', *Characteristics of Social Play* (2008) http://www.education.com/reference/article/characteristics-social-play/

Out to play
• *Start Active, Stay Active*, Department of Health (2011) www.bhfactive.org.uk/userfiles/Documents/startactivestayactive.pdf
— A recent document from the British Heart Foundation reported that a staggering 91 per cent of four year olds are failing to get the recommended daily levels of activity: www.bhfactive.org.uk/beststart
• Mental health implications of outdoor play – Moss (2012)
—*Project Wild Thing*, Green Lions (2013) http://www.thewildnetwork.com/film
• Educational implications – the maths lecturer concerned was Dr Michael Shayer who, with his colleague Dr Philip Adey, published the findings in *Report to the ESRC: Have the norms for volume and heaviness for Year 7 changed since the mid-70's?* (2005) www.researchcatalogue.esrc.ac.uk/grants/RES-000-22-1379/read
• Sir Digby Jones – Graeme Paton, 'The danger from our cottonwool kids', *Daily Telegraph* (7 July 2007) www.telegraph.co.uk/news/uknews/1541803/The-danger-from-our-cotton-wool-kids.html
• Richard Branson story – Branson (2007)
• David Attenborough quote – from an address to the Communicate Conference, *Connecting with Nature*, University of Bristol (November 2010)
• Jesuit quote – attributed to St Ignatius Loyola, among others
• Margaret McMillan quote – circa 1925, no recorded reference

Great minds think alike
• For early years pioneers – see Elkin (2015) and Jarvis, et al (2016)
• Nutbrown Review: *Foundations for Quality*, Professor Cathy Nutbrown (HMSO 2012) https://www.gov.uk/government/uploads/system/uploads/attachment_data/file/175463/Nutbrown-review.pdf

Everything to play for
• 'the imagination is warm and impressions are permanent' – quote from letter by Thomas Jefferson (1785)
• Alison Gopnik quote – 'A Conversation with Dr Alison Gopnik', *NAEYC*, vol. 3, no. 2 (December 2009/January 2010) www.naeyc.org/files/tyc/file/TYC_V3N2_Gopnik.pdf
• Further evidence – Gopnik is by no means alone in her belief that 'pre-school' is an important stage in children's education and all-round development.
—Collette Taylor, 'Learning in early childhood: relationships, experiences and 'learning to be' (2015) http://onlinelibrary.wiley.com/enhanced/doi/10.1111/d.1 2117?elqaid=1452&elqat=2&elqTrackId=2e6192f9148d45d1b73a24e3800c9673

—Dr David Whitebread's summary of the evidence for a later school starting age (2014) www.toomuchtoosoon.org/uploads/2/0/3/8/20381265/school_starting_age_-_the_evidence.pdf

CHAPTER THREE

More background information for this chapter is available in *Toxic Childhood: How the modern world is damaging our children and what we can do about it* (2006 and 2015) In fact, it was while preparing the second edition of *Toxic Childhood* for print that I began to write *Upstart*. By then, I'd realised that the most practical way to counter the 'toxic childhood system' is to ensure the best possible out-of-home care and play-based education for children under the age of seven.

The special needs explosion
• Dyslexia statistics – Dyslexia Research Trust www.dyslexic.org.uk
• ADHD statistics – UK (2014) http://www.nhs.uk/conditions/attention-deficit-hyperactivity-disorder/Pages/Introduction.aspx
    —US http://www.cdc.gov/nchs/fastats/adhd.htm
    —Since 2013 there has been concern about the year-on-year increases in prescriptions for medication such as Ritalin on the principle that, in many cases, simple lifestyle adjustments are more effective than medical interventions. See *NHS News* (11 November 2013) www.nhs.uk/news/2013/11November/Pages/Experts-argue-that-ADHD-is-overdiagnosed.aspx
• ASD statistics
    —American Academy of Pediatrics website www.aap.org/en-us/Pages/Default.aspx (2005)
    —Centre for Disease Control and Prevention (2014) www.cdc.gov/ncbddd/autism/data
• UK autism figures – Office for National Statistics, *Survey of the Mental Health of Children and Young People in Great Britain* (2004)
    —UK National Autistic Society website www.autism.org.uk/About/What-is/Myths-facts-stats
• Dyspraxia – NHS www.nhs.uk/conditions/Dyspraxia-(childhood)/Pages/Introduction.aspx
    —Dyspraxia Foundation www.dyspraxiafoundation.org.uk/about-dyspraxia/

How special is special?
• UNICEF Report – *An overview of child wellbeing in rich countries* (2007) https://www.unicef-irc.org/publications/pdf/rc7_eng.pdf
• 2006 national study of children's language development – *The Cost to the Nation of Children's Poor Communication*, ICAN (2006)
• Children's physical coordination – *Babies, Brains and Balance*, Harborough Sure Start, Leicestershire (2010) www.youtube.com/watch?v=e7lPaZodAkE
    —Sue Learner, 'Pre-school children today have "poorer physical and motor skills than 20 years ago"', *Day Nurseries* (3 September 2014) www.daynurseries.co.uk/news/article.cfm/id/1565027/pre-school-children-poorer-physical-skills-than-20-years-ago
    —Javier Espinoza, 'Nearly half of children "leave [primary] school without basic movement skills", study says', *Daily Telegraph* (24 June 2015) www.telegraph.co.uk/education/educationnews/11693791/Nearly-half-of-children-leave-school-without-basic-movement-skills-study-says.html

Levels of empathy in US college students – Sarah H. Konrath, et al., 'Changes in Dispositional Empathy in American College Students Over Time: A meta-analysis', *Personality and Social Psychology Review* (2011) www.ipearlab.org/media/publications/Changes_in_Dispositional_Empathy_-_Sara_Konrath.pdf

—Jamil Zakri, 'What, Me Care? Young Are Less Empathetic', *Scientific American Mind*, (1 January 2011) www.scientificamerican.com/article/what-me-care/

• 'Sticking plaster solutions' – in 2005, when the government finally noticed the growing incidence of language delay, a training package called Communication Matters was issued to EY providers, including childminders. It was followed in 2008 by another package called *Every Child A Talker*. As children's spoken language skills in disadvantaged areas continued to decline, 2011 was declared 'The Year of Communication'. Unfortunately, by then, there had been a change of government and the Year was poorly publicised, so very few people heard about it.

• Ofsted revision of Special Educational Needs – *SEN and Disability Review* (2010) www.gov.uk/government/publications/special-educational-needs-and-disability-review

—Jeevan Vaasger, 'Half of some special needs children misdiagnosed', *Guardian* (14 September 2010) www.theguardian.com/education/2010/sep/14/half-special-needs-children-misdiagnosed

I ♥ my iPad

• Research on use of iPads by under-twos – Jenny Radesky, et al., 'Mobile and Interactive Media Use by Young Children: The good, the bad and the unknown', *Paediatrics* (January 2015) pediatrics.aappublications.org/content/135/1/1

—Sarah Knapton, 'Using iPads to pacify children may harm their development', *Daily Telegraph* (1 February 2015) www.telegraph.co.uk/news/science/science-news/11382711/Using-iPads-to-pacify-children-may-harm-their-development-say-scientists.html

• Daniel Anderson quote – Dr Victor Strasburger, 'First do no harm: Why have parents and paediatricians missed the boat on children and the media?', *Journal of Paediatrics*, vol. 151, issue 54 (2006)

• More than 70 per cent of UK households owned a tablet in 2014 – since Ofcom reported tablet ownership had trebled in only three years (in 2011 it was 7 per cent), it's likely that tablet use will soon be normal behaviour among almost all families

—Ofcom's survey of Adult Media Use and Attitudes (2015) stakeholders. ofcom.org.uk/binaries/research/media-literacy/media-lit-10years/2015_Adults_media_use_and_attitudes_report.pdf

• Sally Weale, 'A third of pre-school children have their own iPad', *Guardian* (6 October 15) www.theguardian.com/education/2015/oct/06/third-pre-school-children-have-own-ipad-study

• Use by under-ones – Michael Miller, 'Look who's swiping now: 6-month-old babies are using smartphones, study says', *Washington Post* (27 April 2015) www.washingtonpost.com/news/morning-mix/wp/2015/04/27/look-whos-swiping-now-6-month-old-babies-are-using-smartphones-study-says/

• American Academy of Paediatrics advice – www.aap.org/en-us/advocacy-and-policy/aap-health-initiatives/pages/media-and-children.aspx

Junk food and junk play

• Increases in consumption of junk food – Sue Palmer, Chapter 1: Food for Thought, *Toxic Childhood* (2015)

• WHO and obesity – www.who.int/mediacentre/factsheets/fs311/en/
• Child obesity levelling off – 'Child obesity rates are "stabilising"', *NHS Choices* (30 January 2015) www.nhs.uk/news/2015/01January/Pages/Child-obesity-rates-are-stabilising.aspx

Consumerism, concern and control
• The decline of 'real play' has been well catalogued over recent years – see Layard and Dunn (2007), Gill (2007), Palmer (2006, 2015)
• Children not playing out in their neighbourhoods – how lack of outdoor play has become normalised – Rob Wheway, 'Children should be free to play, not prisoners in their own homes', *Guardian* (15 October 2015) www.theguardian.com/housing-network/2015/oct/15/children-free-play-not-prisoners-homes?CMP=Share_iOSApp_Other
• Stephen Moss quote – from a video launching the Natural Childhood Report (August 2012) www.youtube.com/watch?v=rBwKrbfhgDU
    — According to 2016 research: 'Three quarters of UK children spend less time outdoors than prison inmates', Damian Carrington, *Guardian* (25 March 2016)

Normalisation, nature and culture
• Global marketing competition to 'own' children – Shor (2004), Linn (2005), Mayo and Nairn (2009), Palmer (2015)
• UK government report 'The Bailey Review', *Letting Children Be Children*, (2011) www.gov.uk/government/uploads/system/uploads/attachment_data/file/175418/Bailey_Review.pdf
• Campaign for a Commercial-Free Childhood – www.commercialfreechildhood.org/
• Save Childhood Movement – www.savechildhood.net/
• Bye Buy Childhood – www.byebuychildhood.org/
• Prof Gerard Hastings, Professor of Social Marketing, University of Stirling – Personal interview (2012)
• The current approach in the USA and UK – at present the growing body of research on the significance of 'real play' has not been communicated to parents
    —Dr Aric Sigman, 'Child's Play: The new paediatric prescription', *British Association for Community Child Health News*, Annual Scientific Meeting Special Issue (December 2012)

The perils of modern parenting
• Authoritative parenting – although most researchers use the term 'authoritative', the terminology for other parenting styles varies from study to study. I've chosen what seemed to me the simplest, clearest vocabulary for the behaviour involved.
    —See Martin (2005), Lee and Lee (2009)
    —Dr Gwen Dewar, 'The authoritative parenting style: warmth, rationality and high standards', *Parenting Science* (2010) www.parentingscience.com/authoritative-parenting-style.html

Coda
• 2015 government report on CAMHS –There's no doubt among families and clinicians that CAMHS is under severe stress but statistics on child and adolescent mental health are sadly lacking, since there has been no national survey of the under-16 age group since 2005
    —Nick Triggle, 'Child mental health services "face overhaul"', *BBC News*, (17 March 2015) http://www.bbc.co.uk/news/health-31914765

—Mental Health Foundation report: http://www.mentalhealth.org.uk/help-information/mental-health-statistics/children-young-people/)

—At time of writing there is widespread concern among health professionals about the lack of national statistics. See Ami Sedgi, 'What is the state of children's mental health today?', *Guardian* (5 January 2015) www.theguardian.com/society/christmas-charity-appeal-2014-blog/2015/jan/05/-sp-state-children-young-people-mental-health-today

• The significance of childhood play for mental health: see 'The decline of play and the rise in children's mental disorders' by Peter Gray in *Psychology Today* (26 January 2010) www.psychologytoday.com/blog/freedom-learn/201001/the-decline-play-and-rise-in-childrens-mental-disorders Gray's arguments are widely accepted among developmental psychologists and clinicians but, when faced with a distressed child, their attention must inevitably be focused on remediation

CHAPTER FOUR

Tuning into language

• Dr Sally Ward – see Ward (2002) Tragically, Dr Ward died shortly after her book on early language development was published. However, her research helped to convince the government and educational establishment of the significance of early interaction between parent and child

• Clare and David Mills – video, *Too Much Too Young,* is available and still extremely relevant (1998) www.millsproductions.co.uk/early-years/too-much-too-young.shtml

• Dr Ann Locke – Personal interview (2000)

• ICAN report – *The Cost to the Nation of Children's Poor Communication* (ICAN 2006)

Laying the foundations

• The adaptation of the human brain for literacy – Wolf (2008)

Anglo-Saxon attitudes versus Finnish foundations

• Ofsted report – 'The education of six-year-olds in England, Denmark and Finland' (2003) www.educationengland.org.uk/documents/pdfs/2003-ofsted-six-year-olds-comparative.pdf

• Agneta's sentence activity – I've since been told by Finnish Early Years practitioners that this sort of activity isn't necessary if children have time to develop self-regulation skills through their own free play (perhaps Agneta's activity impressed me so much because I have some deeply entrenched Anglo-Saxon attitudes of my own). Nevertheless, the children all obviously enjoyed it, the 'sentence-saying' lasted no more than a minute, and it seemed to me a great way of developing the social and communication skills the children would require in a busy setting. It's lived on in my memory because the contrast with an English circle time was so stark.

Let's hear it for story and song!

• Evolutionary connections between music and language – Mithen (2006)

• Music's role in literacy – see Maria Kay (2013). Kay provides guidance for teachers in using musical activities to lay strong foundations for literacy

• Stories and mental processing – there's an enormous amount of academic literature on this subject but it's very well summarised in Boyd (2009)

• Kieran Egan quote – Egan (2014). As Professor of Education at Simon Fraser University in Canada, Egan has been exploring the significance of narrative in early cognitive development for over thirty years
  —Also www.educ.sfu.ca/kegan/default.html

The little boy who said 'Fish'

• Pie Corbett's work on developing storytelling skills in young children is now well-known in UK schools. We worked together for many years on *Talk for Writing* materials
• 'yuk and wow'– Susan Greenfield, 'We are at risk of losing our imagination' *Guardian* (25 August 2006) www.theguardian.com/education/2006/apr/25/elearning.schools

Nature versus culture

• For more background on this subject – see Donald (2001)
• Simple shortcuts to cognitive development – NICHD Early Child Care Research Network, 'Pathways to Reading: The role of oral language in the transition to reading', *Developmental Psychology* (2005) www.ncbi.nlm.nih.gov/pubmed/15769197
  —The researchers conclude that 'environments rich in language stimulation and conversation will not only build general language skills but will also have the positive consequence of supplementing vocabulary and metalinguistic skills. The reverse is not necessarily true. That is, simply teaching vocabulary and phonemic awareness, although perhaps necessary, would not be sufficient to buttress general language skills.'
• Cutting to the educational chase in literacy – Tony Bertram and Chris Pascal, 'What counts in early learning?', *Contemporary perspectives in early childhood curriculum*, eds., O.N. Saracho and B. Spodek (IAP 2002) This paper identifies three core elements of effective learners: 'dispositions to learn, social competence and self-concept, and social and emotional wellbeing'. The authors argue that a primary focus on subject knowledge, particularly language and mathematical competency, is insufficient.
• Human beings aren't just machines to be programmed – N.C. Paige, G.B. McLaughlin and J.W. Almon, *Reading in Kindergarten: Nothing to gain and much to lose*, Alliance for Childhood (2012) allianceforchildhood.org/sites/allianceforchildhood.org/files/file/Reading_Instruction_in_Kindergarten.pdf
• Phonics – during the 'Primary Wars' in Chapter 1, phonics became a key area of dispute between progressive and traditionalist educators, and ever since politicians have regarded it as critically important in the teaching of reading. The arguments have become polarised, and it is now almost impossible to have a reasoned discussion about phonics. One is immediately seen as either 'for it or against it'

Huckt on fonics

• Over a century of squabbling about phonics – the first recorded account of these squabbles that I've found is in Edmund Huey, *The Psychology and Pedagogy of Reading*, (1908)
• A long-time fan of phonics – my first published phonics course, the Language 1 materials of *The Longman Book Project* (1994), helped to re-establish phonics in literacy teaching after several decades of neglect. I subsequently wrote phonics resources for Scholastic, Ginn, the BBC, Dorling Kindersley and others. *Synthetic*

Phonix Cubes (2005) won a BERA (British Education Research Association) award.

• 'Lucky children' – I wrote the list below in a recent blog. It summarises how, without any teaching at all, many children simply 'pick up' reading and writing through repeated, intrinsically motivating experiences

Daily experiences	How they build sound foundations for literacy	Why they work
Children's self-chosen, active, creative play (as often as possible, outdoors)	All-round bodily coordination and control; visual discrimination; problem-solving skills, and much more...	Play is children's inborn learning drive, and develops their motivation to learn
Moving to music, singing songs, chanting rhymes	Auditory discrimination and memory, and many other abilities that underpin literacy	Music and song come naturally to human beings so they're great fun for children
Opportunities to talk about events/items of interest	Development of spoken language and listening skills	Talk is a key way in which adults pass on knowledge and children consolidate their understanding
Sharing stories and picture books (favourite ones over and over again)	Vocabulary development, auditory memory and listening skills, familiarity with narrative patterns, understanding of 'how books work'	We are 'a storying animal' so children love stories – and sharing them with beloved adults is a deeply satisfying emotional experience
Opportunities for mark-making, painting, drawing, etc.	Motor control, hand–eye coordination, symbolic representation	Children long to communicate and make their mark on the world
Opportunities to see adults reading and writing **by hand**, for real-life purposes	Understanding of why literacy is important in daily life, and how it's done	Mimicry is a vital learning drive. Children copy the behaviour of the adults they love and admire

• Tried and tested activities to develop literacy skills – Palmer and Bayley (2013)
• Six-year-old phonics test – In 2015, an Open Letter outlining many objections to this test and calling for its abolition was sent to the Secretary of State for Education. It was signed by distinguished academics, the Chairs of major educational associations and the General Secretary of the National Association of Headteachers. The Education Secretary ignored it
   —www.gov.uk/government/publications/key-stage-1-assessment-and-reporting-arrangements-ara/phonics-screening-check

—www.opnlttr.com/letter/open-letter-michael-gove-why-year-1-phonics-check-must-go

• Quote from Minister for Schools – Nick Gibb, 'There's no excuse for children leaving primary school unable to read', *Guardian* (25 September 2014) www.theguardian.com/teacher-network/teacher-blog/2014/sep/25/primary-school-children-read-phonics

More haste, less success

• Academic arguments against current policy – as well as evidence-based arguments from UK experts, such as contributors to the Alexander Report (see Chapter 1) and Margaret Clark (below), two research reviews were recently published in the USA, where children are subjected to a similar regime

—Lillian C. Katz, *Lively Minds: Distinctions between intellectual and academic goals for young childre*n, University of Illinois (DEY 2015) deyproject.files.wordpress.com/2015/04/dey-lively-minds-4-8-15.pdf

—Nancy Carlton Paige, et al., *Reading Instruction in Kindergarten: Little to gain and much to lose*, Alliance for Childhood (2015) www.allianceforchildhood.org/sites/allianceforchildhood.org/files/file/Reading_Instruction_in_Kindergarten.pdf

• Dr Margaret Clark – Dr Clark, a highly respected literacy academic, offers a balanced critique, raising not only the unreliability of the test but also the escalating costs of this annual procedure. The government has, at time of writing, not responded

—'Evidence-Based Critique on Synthetic Phonics in Literacy Learning', *Primary First* (2015) also via the United Kingdom Literacy Association ukla.org/downloads/M_Clark_Primary_First_Article_on_synthetic_phonics_1.pdf See also, Clark, 2016

• Research in New Zealand – Sebastian P. Suggate, Elizabeth A. Schaughency and Elaine Reese, 'Children learning to read later catch up to children reading earlier', *Early Childhood Research Quarterly*, 28 (2013) web.uvic.ca/~gtreloar/Articles/Language Arts/Children learning to read later catch up to children reading earlier.pdf

• Sad little anecdote – I heard this story from the researcher concerned

• European research on handwriting – research conducted by Dr József Nagy of Attila Jozsef University in Hungary. He describes it in the *Too Much Too Young* video, referenced in 'Tuning in to language' above, but, since I don't speak Hungarian, I've been unable to track down a written reference

The third R

• Panic about maths – the phenomenon of 'maths anxiety' is well documented, for example in Sarah Sparks, 'Summary', 'Researchers Probe Causes of Math Anxiety', *Education Week* (16 May 2011) www.edweek.org/ew/articles/2011/05/18/31math_ep.h30.html

• Sound developmental principles – for an introduction to 'number sense' for early years teachers see Jenni Black, *Early Number Sense*, Enriching Mathematics, University of Cambridge (2014) nrich.maths.org/10737

• The significance of play in early maths – see a report of a symposium held at John Curtin University, Fremantle, Western Australia by Professor Janette Bobis and Sue Dockett et al., *Playing with Mathematics: Play in early childhood as a context for mathematical learning* (2010)

• Learning through play is time well spent – see Gerardo Ramires, et al., 'Maths Anxiety, Working Memory, and Math Achievement in Early Elementary School', *Journal of Cognition and Development,* 14:2 (2013)

—Ramires claims problems become apparent in first grade (age six) and 'lead to a snowball effect that exerts an increasing cost on math achievement by changing students' attitudes and motivational approaches towards math avoidance, and ultimately reducing math competence'

Maths, motivation and meaning

• Cognitively Guided Instruction – I'm indebted to Lio Moscardino of the University of Strathclyde for the opportunity to attend a seminar on CGI and talk with students who are using the strategy in the classroom. See Carpenter, et al. (2014)

• Video footage of Hungarian kindergarten – this was a full-length recording of a lesson which presumably ended up on the cutting-room floor. Hungarian maths results – featured in David Mills, *Too Much Too Young*. See 'Tuning in to language' above

Coda

• Teenagers failing to achieve Grade C – see report (August 2015) www.gov.uk/government/news/summer-2015-gcse-results-a-brief-explanation

• Mental health problems mushrooming – see Notes for Chapter 3 and Chapter 5

CHAPTER FIVE

• Choose well-educated, high-income parents – Colin Richards, 'Educational Achievement in English Primary Education', *Education 3-13: International Journal of Primary, Elementary and Early Years Education* (2008) www.tandfonline.com/doi/full/10.1080/03004270801959239

—Archer (2002)

• Be female – until the introduction of state education girls had less access to education than boys so inevitably trailed behind. Since then they have consistently out-performed boys from the early stages, starting with literacy and, of recent years, across the board

—See *Gender and Education: The evidence on pupils in England*, DfES (2007) webarchive.nationalarchives.gov.uk/20130401151715/http://www.education.gov. uk/publications/eOrderingDownload/00389-2007BKT-EN.pdf

• Adjustment of marking systems – Linda Croxford, et al., 'Gender and Pupil Performance: Where do the problems lie?', *Scottish Educational Review* (2003) www.scotedreview.org.uk/media/scottish-educational-review/articles/171.pdf

• Don't be a summerborn – Elizabeth Sykes, et al., *Birthdate Effects: A review of literature from 1990 on*, Cambridge Assessment, (February 2009) www. cambridgeassessment.org.uk/images/109784-birthdate-effects-a-review-of-the-literature-from-1990-on.pdf

• In 2016, the UK ranked 25th out of 37 wealthy countries on a UNICEF survey of the gap in educational and health outcomes between rich and poor – 'UK lags behind other rich countries in child inequality' Hannah Richardson, BBC online, 14 April 2016

PART ONE: RICH AND POOR

• Oxfam report 2014 – Sarah Dransfield, *A Tale of Two Britains: Inequality in the UK*, Oxfam (2014) www.oxfam.org.uk/blogs/2014/03/5-richest-families-in-uk-are-wealthier-than-poorest-20-pc

• Erzsebet Bukodi, John Goldthorpe, et al., 'The mobility problem in Britain: new

findings from the analysis of birth cohorts', *British Journal of Sociology* (March 2015) onlinelibrary.wiley.com/enhanced/doi/10.1111/1468-4446.12096/
• Quote from Dr John Goldthorpe – University of Oxford press release (11 June 2014) www.spi.ox.ac.uk/about-us/announcements/item/social-mobility-has-not-stalled-but-more-of-us-are-heading-down-the-social-ladder.html
• Statistics on child poverty in the UK – Barnardos www.barnardos.org.uk/what_we_do/our_work/child_poverty/child_poverty_what_is_poverty/child_poverty_statistics_facts.htm
• Report on the growing divide between rich and poor – *The Greatest Divide*, Fabian Society (December 2015) www.fabians.org.uk/wp-content/uploads/2015/12/The-Greatest-Divide-new.pdf

Ethics and economics
• Inequality is bad for everyone – Wilkinson and Pickett (2010)
• Eradicating child poverty by 2020 – Tony Blair, 'Pledge to eliminate child poverty' *BBC News* (18 March 1999) news.bbc.co.uk/1/hi/uk_politics/298745. stm For many people in education and children's services (including me), this was an inspirational aim, which convinced us to participate in New Labour's massive programme of reforms
• James Heckman quote – The 'Heckman Equation' reduced a complex social (and human) problem to figures on a balance sheet. See '4 Big Benefits of Investing in Early Childhood Developments', *Heckman* (21 January 2015) heckmanequation. org/content/4-big-benefits-investing-early-childhood-development
• Mushrooming workloads and mountains of bureaucracy – see my description of this period in *21st Century Boys* (2008), when the madness was at its height: 'The UK government has invested billions of pounds to eradicate child poverty, and devised innumerable... strategies and initiatives for the purpose, with targets, outcome duties, league tables and tick lists galore. And since 1997 well over half a million children have indeed been technically transferred from one side of a poverty balance sheet to the other. Sadly, out in the real world it's gradually become clear that the change happened only on paper: poor children's lives had not got noticeably better.' By summer 2008 a *Guardian* columnist was complaining that 'Evidence, reality, consequences, the classroom failures of struggling pupils - none of these matter. The statistics, however flawed and unreliable, are all that count'.
• Family Nurse Partnership – this project (known as the Nurse Family Partnership in the USA) was devised by Professor David Olds in Colorado in the 1970s, and was probably highly influenced by the UK's recent introduction of health visitors. Due to the personal connections forged between nurse and family, it's been one of the most successful projects for improving poor children's early nurture, and was brought back to the UK, to be used specifically for 'at-risk' young families http://fnp.nhs.uk
• The significance of ongoing support – Leon Feinstein, 'Very Early Evidence', *Centrepiece*, Summer (2003) intouniversity.org/sites/all/files/userfiles/files/Leon Feinstein evidence fro early years.pdf
• Richard Layard quote – Palmer, 2008

A tale of under-achievement?
• Sally Ward's research – see Chapter 4 (page 75)
• Hart-Risley research – Hart and Risley (1995) and Summary, Rice University

literacy.rice.edu/thirty-million-word-gap. In the early 1990s, Betty Hart and Todd Risley followed three groups of children through the early years of childhood, from 'professional', 'working-class' and 'welfare' families. They regularly tape-recorded hour-long periods of interaction between adults and children in their homes, analysed the findings and extrapolated how many different words the various children had heard, in conversations with adults, by the age of four. On average, it appeared a professional's child has heard around 50 million words, a working-class child 30 million and a welfare child a meagre 12 million. To ram home the alarming difference in language exposure, they found that, by the age of three, the average vocabulary level of professional children was higher than that of the *parents* in the welfare group.

• Discouraging versus encouraging language – Hart and Risley (1995) Hart and Risley didn't just measure the number of words children heard and spoke. They also recorded differences in the way children were spoken to, and the extent to which parents explained things, gave choices or listened to what they had to say. By the age of three, professional children had heard about 700,000 encouragements and only 80,000 discouragements. In contrast, the welfare child had been encouraged only 60,000 times and discouraged 120,000. Working-class children were somewhere in the middle.

• Developing language skills – Myae Han, et al., 'Does Play Make a Difference? How Play Intervention Affects the Vocabulary Learning of At-Risk Preschoolers', *American Journal of Play* (Summer 2010) www.journalofplay.org/sites/www. journalofplay.org/files/pdf-articles/3-1-article-does-play-make-a-difference. pdf

• 'Readiness' for education of children in early-start countries – Findings from Bradbury, et al., *Inequality during the Early Years: Child outcomes and readiness to learn in Australia, Canada, United Kingdom and United States,* Institute for the Study of Labor, Discussion Paper No. 6120 (Bonn 2011) ftp.iza.org/dp6120.pdf This report found the poorest outcomes were in the USA and UK; Canada, which doesn't start school till six and has a less 'schoolified' approach to early learning had the best outcomes; Australia, which had a similarly laid-back approach until recently, came second.

A tale of dwindling achievement

• Abecdarian project – http://abc.fpg.unc.edu/

• Fan of Direct Instruction – Shepard Barbash, 'Pre-K *Can* Work', *City Journal,* Autumn (2008) www.city-journal.org/2008/18_4_pre-k.html

• The few longitudinal studies available – See Notes, Chapter 4, 'Huckt on Phonics' regarding Lilian Katz, *Lively Minds* (2015) via Valerie Strauss, 'Report debunks "earlier is better" academic instruction for young children', *Washington Post* (12 April 2015) www.washingtonpost.com/news/answer-sheet/wp/2015/04/12/ report-debunks-earlier-is-better-academic-instruction-for-young-children/

• 2002 US longitudinal study – R. A. Marcon, 'Moving Up the Grades: Relationships between preschool model and later school success', *Early Childhood Research and Practice* (2002) ecrp.uiuc.edu/v4n1/marcon.html

• Resilience – Harvard Centre for the Developing Child developingchild.harvard. edu/science/key-concepts/resilience/

• Conflict between early academic teaching and social and emotional development —C. Blair, 'School Readiness: 'Integration of cognition and emotion in a

neurobiological conceptualization of child functioning at school entry', *American Psychologist*, 57.2 (2002) www.ncbi.nlm.nih.gov/pubmed/11899554
• Significance of early social and emotional development in long-term resilience – Damon E. Jones, et al., 'Early Social and Emotional Functioning and Public Health: The relationship between kindergarten social competence and future wellness', *American Journal of Public Health*, (15 July 2015) ajph.aphapublications.org/doi/pdf/10.2105/AJPH.2015.302630

Misreading the evidence

• High/Scope Perry Project – see Notes, Chapter 4, 'Nature versus culture'. The allocation of children to the three groups described in *Upstart* is also described by Paige (2012) and Katz (2015). However, in official High/Scope publications, reference is made to only two groups: one on the High/Scope programme and one that was not. See www.highscope.org/content.asp?contentid=219 This isn't surprising, as the High/Scope Foundation has a programme to sell and the suggestion that 'free play' may be similarly effective would not be helpful.
• TV interview about High/Scope with David Weikart – in this interview, the three groups are clearly described and Weikart makes it clear that it was children in the formal group who suffered serious long-term deleterious social and emotional effects. See *Panorama*, (late 1990s), clip www.youtube.com/watch?v=BlfJMFtHjbw
• Long tail of underachievement – composed of children from economically deprived backgrounds: the same is true in the USA, despite some extreme examples of schoolification and drilling of four to seven year olds. See Valerie Strauss, 'Why forcing kids to do things "sooner and faster" doesn't get them further in school', *Washington Post* (11 January 2016) www.washingtonpost.com/news/answer-sheet/wp/2016/01/11/why-forcing-kids-to-do-things-sooner-and-faster-doesn't-get-them-further-in-school/

Smart-arsed, selfish and smug

• Empathy research – see Jamil Zaki, 'What, Me Care? Young Are Less Empathetic', *Scientific American* (1 January 2011) www.scientificamerican.com/article/what-me-care/ It refers to a research study by Sarah Konrath at the University of Mitchigan
—For more detail on the significance of empathy see de Waal (2007) and Rifkin (2009)
—Also RSAnimate video summing up Rifkin's theory www.thersa.org/events/rsaanimate/animate/rsa-animate-the-empathic-civilisation
• Entitlement research – Douglas Quenga, 'Seeing Narcissim Everywhere', *New York Times* (5 August 2013) regarding research by Professor Jean Twenge of San Diego State University www.nytimes.com/2013/08/06/science/seeing-narcissists-everywhere.html
—Twenge (2009)
• Employers' complaints about graduate recruits – Staff Writers, 'Common Complaints Employers have about Recent Grads', *Online College* (10 September 2012) www.onlinecollege.org/2012/09/10/13-common-complaints-employers-have-about-recent-grads/
—Jess Denham, 'Graduates unprepared for employment', *Independent* (13 September 2013) www.independent.co.uk/student/graduates-unprepared-for-employment-8814643.html

Poor little rich kids

• Jamie Downward, 'Emotional health in childhood is the key to future happiness', *Observer* (8 November 2014)
 —*The Causes and Effects of Wellbeing*, LSE Centre for Economic Performance cep.lse.ac.uk/_new/research/wellbeing/causes_and_effects_of_wellbeing.asp
• Teachers' concern about mental health of wealthy pupils – Sian Griffiths, 'Top schools face mental health crisis', *Sunday Times* (4 October 2015)
• The 'teacher from a posh prep school' would prefer to remain anonymous
• Quote from MD of educational consultancy and other details about nursery hothousing: Tanith Carey, 'The Race for Nursery Places', *Daily Telegraph* (28 May 2015) www.telegraph.co.uk/women/mother-tongue/11632773/The-race-for-nursery-places.html
• Quote about six-year-old boy under pressure – Sally Jones, 'Tutoring: avoiding hothousing', *School House Magazine* (2015) www.schoolhousemagazine.co.uk/education/tutoring/tutoring-avoiding-hothousing
• Long-term study of 'intelligent and good learners' – see Notes, Chapter 1, 'The Longevity Project'

Coda

• UNICEF World Happiness Report (most recent 2015) worldhappiness.report/

PART TWO: BOYS AND GIRLS

• Since 2004, I have researched two books on the effects of modern life on boys' and girls' development, *21st Century Boys* (2009) and *21st Century Girls* (2013). Both argue that gender stereotyping, driven by contemporary culture, affects the educational and life trajectories of both sexes from the moment of birth.
• Sumerian schoolboy – 'Sumerian School Days [Text and Object]', *Children and Youth History*, Item #408 (accessed 22 December 2015) chnm.gmu.edu/cyh/primary-sources/408
• Shakespeare reference – from *As You Like It*
• Wordsworth reference – from 'Intimations of Immortality'
• Gender gap a global phenomenon – girls' higher achievement happens, of course, only in countries where they are are given equal access to education with boys, which in many parts of the world is not the case.
• Late-start countries doing better – George Arnett, 'Gender equality report: not one country has fully closed the gap yet', *Guardian* (28 October 2014) www.theguardian.com/news/datablog/2014/oct/28/not-one-country-has-fully-closed-gender gap-yet-report-shows 'Gender differences in Scholastic Achievement : A Meta-Analysis' Voyer D and Voyer SD in *Psychological Bulletin*, Vol 140:4 (2014) https://www.apa.org/pubs/journals/releases/bul-a0036620.pdf
• Gap reverses in employment – Julia Kollewe, 'Gender pay gap: women effectively working for free until the end of the year', *Guardian* (9 November 2014) www.theguardian.com/world/2015/nov/09/gender-pay-gap-women-working-free-until-end-of-year

Nature, nurture and gender

• Steve Connor, 'Girls have been faster learners for six million years', *Independent* 15 April 2004

• Nature article – E. V. Lonsdorf, L.E. Eberley, A.E. Pusey, 'Sex differences in learning in chimpanzees', *Nature 428* (2004)
• Gender as 'a cultural concept' over the last fifty years – Palmer (2008 and 2013)
• Male development delay – Biddulph (1998) and Eliot (2010)

The trouble with gender

• Elizabeth Spelke quote – from a debate on 'The Science of Gender and Science – Pinker vs Spelke', *The Edge*, online (16 May 2005) edge.org/event/the-science-of-gender-and-science-pinker-vs-spelke-a-debate
• Variation in behaviour between/within gender categories – for example Diane F. Halpern, *Sex Differences in Cognitive Abilities,* 4th ed., Psychology Press (2011)
• Children's awareness of gender as a permanent characteristic – Dr Robin Banerjee, 'Gender development', *OpenLearn,* Open University (2005) www.open.edu/openlearn/body-mind/childhood-youth/early-years/gender-development
• Commercial gender stereotyping of children and the effects of modern lifestyles on child-rearing – for more detailed information see Palmer (2008 and 2013)

The trouble with boys

• Latest Foundation Stage Profile statistics – Sally Weale, 'Boys trail in literacy and numeracy when starting school', *Guardian* (13 October 2015) www.theguardian.com/education/2015/oct/13/boys-trail-girls-literacy-numeracy-when-starting-school
• Female/male graduates – this was first noticed in 2011. See Graeme Paton, 'David Willetts warns about "striking" university gender gap', *Daily Telegraph* (6 November 2011) www.telegraph.co.uk/education/universityeducation/8873031/David-Willetts-warns-over-striking-university-gender-gap.html
 —An influx of male students from overseas has evened up gender distribution at universities since 2011 – David Matthews, 'Men in higher education: the figures don't look good, guys', *Times Higher Education Supplement* (6 March 2014) www.timeshighereducation.com/news/men-in-higher-education-the-numbers-dont-look-good-guys/2011807.article
 —However, the gender gap in UK-born students continues to grow – Javier Espinoza, 'Gender gap at universities widens, figures show', *Daily Telegraph* (16 December 2015) www.telegraph.co.uk/education/educationnews/12054756/Gender-gap-at-university-widens-figures-show.html
• Special educational needs – see 'Chapter 1: The Fragile Male', Palmer (2009) for statistics and discussion of gender disparity
• Issues around masculinity – Wilson (2007)
• 'peer police' – this term was coined by Gary Wilson, with whom I've been fortunate to work on many occasions. See www.garywilsonraisingboysachievement.co.uk/
• British Medical Association figures – *Child and Adolescent Mental Health: A guide for healthcare professionals* (2006) – the web reference has been removed

...and the trouble with girls

• Sammi Timimi quote – personal interview (2008)
• Rise in girls' mental health problems – Smitha Mundasad, 'Girls face "sharp rise" in emotional problems', *BBC News* (20 April 2015) www.bbc.co.uk/news/health-32350566
• Jenni Hope, 'One in ten teenage girls has an eating disorder and boys as young as ten are at risk', *Daily Mail,* (20 May 2013) www.dailymail.co.uk/news/article-2328072/Anorexia-One-teenage-girls-eating-disorder-boys-young-risk.html

• 20% of fifteen year olds self-harming – Lorenzo Bacino, 'Shock figures show extent of self-harm in English teenagers', *Guardian* (21 May 2014) www.theguardian.com/society/2014/may/21/shock-figures-self-harm-england-teenagers
• Recent books about gender: Natasha Walter, *Living Dolls* (2010) and Kat Banyard, *The Equality Illusion* (2010)

The power to please
• No evidence that girls/boys are cleverer – Eliot (2010)
• 'More prodigies, more idiots' quote – Steven Pinker on Pinker/Spelke debate. See 'The trouble with gender' www.youtube.com/watch?v=-Hb3oe7-PJ8
• One tiny difference: on girls' potential to make eye contact – Leeb and Gillian, 'Here's looking at you, kid! A longitudinal study of perceived gender differences in mutual gaze behaviour in young infants', *Sex Roles*, 50: 1–14 (2004)
• Girls' imitation of friendly facial expressions at six months, earlier language skills and social gesturing – Eliot (2010)

Good girls and naughty boys
• Twelve-month-old girls four times as likely to check for maternal approval – Leeb and Gillian (as above)
• Adults deterring girls from active physical play – Emily R. Mondschein, Karen E. Adolph, and Catherine S. Tamis-LeMonda, 'Gender bias in mothers' expectations about infant crawling', *Journal of Experimental Child Psychology*, 77: 304-16 (2000)
• 'Better a broken bone than a broken spirit'– attributed to Lady Allen of Hurtwood and now the slogan of Play Wales

Coda
• Global Gender Gap index reports.weforum.org/global-gender-gap-report-2014/

CHAPTER SIX

Right from the start
• Development of Finnish early years education and care (ECEC) system – Katja Forssén, Anne-Mari Laukkanen and Veli-Matti Ritakallio, *Policy: The Case of Finland,* Department of Social Policy, University of Turku for the "Welfare Policy and Employment in the Context of Family Change" project meeting, Utrecht (9–10 October 2003)
• OECD quote – from *Babies and Bosses: Reconciling Work and Family Life*, Vol. 4, OECD Publishing (27 May 2005)
• Finnish Baby Box – Helena Lee, 'Why Finnish babies sleep in cardboard boxes', *BBC News* (4 June 2013) www.bbc.co.uk/news/magazine-22751415
• Charges for Day Care/taxation – my information came from my Finnish hosts but the basics are outlined on *Expat Finland* www.expat-finland.com/living_in_finland/.html
• Record in various social factors – see Notes for Chapter 1, 'More Haste, More Problems'
• Entitlement reduced – this paragraph from an email by an early years expert clarifies the change: 'At the moment all children under school age have a subjective right to ECEC. The government is trying to limit the subjective right to ECEC where at least one parent is at home (if the parent is unemployed or on parental

leave for example). This means that in the future the subjective right to ECEC for all children would be 20 hours per week. If the parent is working full-time, the child is granted full-time ECEC. And, if there are extenuating circumstances like family problems, personal difficulties or developmental issues, the child could be granted the right to full-time day care.'

Time and space to play

• Information in this section is based on notes made at the time and checked by my guide, Kaisu Muuronen. Kaisu is an expert in early child development and child protection who works for Child Welfare and Federation of Professional Social Talent Association in Helsinki. We were introduced through the Finnish branch of the Organisation Mondiale pour l'Education Prescolaire (OMEP) – i.e. the World Organisation for Early Childhood

• Adult:child ratio – if/when the ratio is changed it will be one early years teacher and two other practitioners to every 24 children

• Explicit learning targets in the UK – It's now normal practice in both the UK and USA to remind children regularly of their specific 'learning targets'. I've regularly heard comments from England such as this: 'Before they start any written work, all children in our school have to copy the target down off the board. Some of them can hardly write anyway, so they're still copying when the lesson finishes.' Also a Scottish mum recently told me that her five-year-old daughter had brought home a jotter labelled 'My Journey to Level One'.

A tale of two systems

• The requirements for preschool providers in England are set out in the Foundation Stage Framework and monitored by Ofsted inspections – for 2014 requirements see www.gov.uk/government/uploads/system/uploads/attachment_data/file/335504/ EYFS_framework_from_1_September_2014__with_clarification_note.pdf

—Although the maximum child:adult ratio is 13:1 at nursery age, when children enter the reception class it becomes the official pupil:teacher ratio of 30:1, although in most schools a teaching assistant is also employed. When children are five or six, they enter Year 1, and follow the National Curriculum for Key Stage 1

—See www.gov.uk/government/publications/national-curriculum-in-england-framework-for-key-stages-1-to-4

The Finnish ECEC curriculum quoted is the one in use during my visit – www.thl.fi/documents/605877/747474/vasu_english.pdf

—The update to be published in 2016, is the last document in a national curriculum review which has introduced a Pre-Primary Curriculum for children aged six. At time of writing this wasn't available in English. See Notes, Chapter 6, 'Now we are six'. Finnish staffing requirements can be found in this EU document www. europarl.europa.eu/RegData/etudes/etudes/join/2013/495867/IPOL-CULT_ ET(2013)495867(ANN01)_EN.pdf

• 2012 recommendations for changes to qualifications in England – Professor Cathy Nutbrown, *Foundations for Quality: The independent review of early education and childcare qualifications* (June 2012) www.gov.uk/government/uploads/system/ uploads/attachment_data/file/175463/Nutbrown-Review.pdf

• Nutbrown Review suggestions ignored – Catherine Gaunt, 'Nutbrown Level 3 recommendations dismissed', *Nursery World*, (24 March 2014) www.

nurseryworld.co.uk/nursery-world/news/1142905/exclusive-nutbrown-level-recommendations-dismissed
• Attitudes to inspection and national tests in Finland are covered in a government document, *Finnish Education in a Nutshell*
• www.minedu.fi/export/sites/default/OPM/Julkaisut/2013/liitteet/Finnish_education_in_a_nuttshell.pdf

Indoor time and space
• Another difference between Finland and the UK is that Mothers Day is in May

Caring communities
• Absences from subsidised nursery attendance in England – 'Evaluation Article – The Common Inspection Framework: Personal development, behaviour and welfare', *Attendance Matters Magazine* (04 September 2015) www.attendancemattersmagonline.co.uk/index.php/component/k2/item/151236-evaluation-article-the-common-inspection-framework-personal-development-behaviour-and-welfare
• Research on the significance of parent–teacher relationships – a research review was published in 2011. See Janet Goodall, et al., *Review of Best Practice in Parental Engagement*, Institute of Education (September 2011)
• Insistence on regular attendance – while there have as yet been no high-profile cases related to preschool attendance, the current regulations have caused many disputes between parents and schools
    —Press Association report, 'More parents in England prosecuted for taking children out of school', *Guardian* (12 August 2015) www.theguardian.com/education/2015/aug/12/increase-parents-england-prosecuted-taking-children-out-of-school
• Pre-primary year in Finland – my Finnish hosts explained these practical details

Now we are six
    The pre-primary year became compulsory in September 2015. For details of the curriculum see www.oph.fi/download/153504_national_core_curriculum_for_pre-primary_education_2010.pdf

Patterns and sounds
    An article about the use of music in early years – based on my first visit to Finland in 2004 www.educationscotland.gov.uk/earlyyearsmatters/t/genericcontent_tcm4674183.asp

Talking teaching
• Risk assessment forms for preschool excursions in UK – over the last two decades, parental anxiety (see Chapter 3), fears of litigation and a general growth in public service paperwork led to massive increases in the documentation required for risk assessment. By 2011, bureaucracy had reached such heights that many schools and settings more or less abandoned out-of-school trips. A culture of risk aversion still lingers in UK education, and the myths remain widespread. The Health and Safety Executive published *School trips and outdoor learning activities: tackling the health and safety myths* (2011) www.hse.gov.uk/services/education/school-trips.pdf

What? Even the Finns?

• Pasi Sahlberg has been a teacher, teacher educator and policy advisor in Finland. He is currently Visiting Professor of Practice at Harvard's Graduate School of Education
— See Sahlberg (2012).
— Also Sahlberg, *The Secret of Finland's Success: Educating Teachers*, Stanford Centre for Opportunity Policy in Education (2010) edpolicy.stanford.edu/sites/default/files/publications/secret-finland%E2%80%99s-success-educating-teachers.pdf

Old and new literacies

• Millions of pounds on updating technology – £550 million pounds in 2013 and estimated to be increasing, despite education cuts. See Richard Vaughan, 'Schools say yes to tablet computers as ICT spending soars', *Times Educational Supplement*, (20 September 2013) www.tes.co.uk/article.aspx?storycode=6358755
• OECD report – Sean Coughlan, 'Computers do not improve pupil results, says OECD', *BBC News* (15 September 2015) www.bbc.co.uk/news/business-34174796
• Stirrings of concern – David Neild, 'Is technology in the classroom good for children?', *Guardian* (24 November 2015) www.theguardian.com/sustainable-business/2015/dec/24/is-technology-in-the-classroom-good-for-children
• A report for ECEC providers – 'Facing the Screen Dilemma: Young children, technology and early education', *Alliance of Childhood* (2013) www.commercialfreechildhood.org/screendilemma
• Neil Postman quotes – Postman (1994)

Coda

• Attempts to emulate Finland's success must start from bottom up – Adam Taylor, '26 Amazing Facts About Finland's Educational System', *Business Insider* (14 December 2011) www.businessinsider.com/finland-education-school-2011-12?op=1&IR=T

CHAPTER SEVEN

Why Upstart?

• Seminar about resilience – *Dangerous Conversation: The impact of Scottish culture on children's resilience*, Edinburgh (13 June 2014)

Joining up the dots

• Recent evidence relating to the decline of play – Peter Gray, 'Give childhood back to children: If we want our offspring to have happy, productive and moral lives, we must allow more time for play, not less', *Independent* (22 January 2014) www.independent.co.uk/voices/comment/give-childhood-back-to-children-if-we-want-our-offspring-to-have-happy-productive-and-moral-lives-we-9054433.html
—Peter Gray, 'K and Preschool Teachers: Last stand in the war on childhood?', *Psychology Today* (8 August 2015) www.psychologytoday.com/blog/freedom-learn/201507/k-preschool-teachers-last-stand-in-war-childhood
—Angela Hanscombe, 'The decline of play in pre-schoolers and the rise in sensory issues', *Washington Post* (1 September 2015) www.washingtonpost.com/news/answer-sheet/wp/2015/09/01/the-decline-of-play-in-preschoolers-and-the-rise-in-sensory-issues/

—'All party group calls for play to be at the heart of "whole child" child health strategy', Policy for Play (13 October 2015) policyforplay.com/2015/10/13/all-party-group-puts-play-at-the-heart-of-proposed-child-health-strategy/

—'Never in my wildest dreams could I have imagined that we would have to defend children's right to play' – quote from a speech by Professor Nancy Carlsson-Paige

—Valerie Strauss, 'How twisted early childhood has become, from a child development expert', *Washington Post* (24 November 2015) www.washingtonpost.com/news/answer-sheet/wp/2015/11/24/how-twisted-early-childhood-education-has-become-from-a-child-development-expert/

• Recent evidence relating to child and adolescent mental health problems – Laura Donelly, 'Children as young as five suffering from depression', *Daily Telegraph* (30 September 2013) www.telegraph.co.uk/news/health/news/10342447/Children-as-young-as-five-suffering-from-depression.html

—Written submission to Parliamentary Select Committee on Health Inquiry by Public Health England (18 March 2014) data.parliament.uk/writtenevidence/committeeevidence.svc/evidencedocument/health-committee/childrens-and-adolescent-mental-health-and-camhs/written/7562.html

—Ami Sedgi, 'What is the state of children's mental health today?', *Guardian* (5 January 2015) www.theguardian.com/society/christmas-charity-appeal-2014-blog/2015/jan/05/-sp-state-children-young-people-mental-health-today

—Judith Walsh, 'Children's mental health is parents' greatest concern', *BBC News* (7 January 2015) www.bbc.co.uk/news/education-30701591

—Judith Burns, 'More pupils have mental health issues, say school staff', *BBC News* (28 May 2015) www.bbc.co.uk/news/education-32075251

—Hannah Richardson, 'Pupils' mental health tops head teachers' concerns', *BBC News* (20 July 2015) www.bbc.co.uk/news/education-33566813

• Recent evidence relating to disadvantaged children's educational failure – two reports referenced in Chapter 5, 'More haste, less success'

—Katz, *Lively Minds* (2015)

—Carlsson-Paige, et al., *Reading Instruction in Kindergarten: Little to gain and much to lose*, DEY Project (13 January 2015)

—Valerie Strauss, 'Why pushing kids to learn too much too soon is counter-productive', *Washington Post* (17 August 2014) www.washingtonpost.com/news/answer-sheet/wp/2015/08/17/why-pushing-kids-to-learn-too-much-too-soon-is-counterproductive/

—Valerie Strauss, 'The kindergarten testing mess', (6 June 2015) www.washingtonpost.com/news/answer-sheet/wp/2015/06/06/the-kindergarten-testing-mess/

—Damon E. Jones PhD, et al., 'Early Social and Emotional Functioning and Public Health: The relationship between kindergarten social competence and future wellness', *American Journal of Public Health*, online (15 July 2015) ajph.aphapublications.org/doi/pdf/10.2105/AJPH.2015.302630

—First educational comparison between early-start and late-start countries — Thomas Dee and Hans Henrik Sievertsen, *The Gift of Time? School Starting Age and Mental Health*, NBER Working Paper No. 21610, US National Bureau of Economic Research (October 2015) cepa.stanford.edu/sites/default/files/WP15-08.pdf

• *Read, Write, Count* Scottish government drive –Read, Write, Count', Scottish

Government website (17 August 2015) news.scotland.gov.uk/News/Read-Write-Count-1c04.aspx

—There's an excellent parents' website: www.readwritecount.scot/ – My concern with this drive is the introduction of testing at five, which will inevitably increase parental anxiety and affect educational practice.

NUT research review – Professor Merryn Hutchins, *Exam Factories*, NUT (June 2015) www.teachers.org.uk/files/exam-factories.pdf

Controversy about baseline testing – The rationale underpinning England's 'basement assessment' system was comprehensively demolished at an academic conference at Newman University, Birmingham (24 February 2016) (see proceedings at www.newman.ac.uk/24feb) so on 7 April 2016 the government quietly abandoned it. However, they did not abandon the policy so another system will undoubtedly follow.

The paradigm trap

• International statistics – since these reviews began, the western countries that have done best in terms of education are ones where school starts later than the UK (in the most recent large-scale review, the 2013 PISA survey, the UK failed to reach the top twenty in any subject). Among the nations that outperformed us, five (Leichtenstein, Estonia, Poland, Switzerland and Finland) start school at seven. See www.oecd.org/pisa/keyfindings/PISA-2012-results-snapshot-Volume-I-ENG.pdf

• OECD review – Sean Coughlan, 'Asia tops biggest global school rankings', *BBC News* (13 May 2015) www.bbc.co.uk/news/business-32608772

• Thomas Dee and Hans Henrik Sievertsen, *The Gift of Time* — see 'Joining up the dots' above

• ADHD most prevalent childhood mental health condition – *Summary Health Statistics for US Children*, National Health Interview Survey (2012) www.cdc.gov/nchs/data/series/sr_10/sr10_258.pdf

• UK prescriptions for Ritalin, etc. – Daniel Boffey, 'Prescriptions for Ritalin and other ADHD drugs double in a decade', *Guardian* (15 August 2015) www.theguardian.com/society/2015/aug/15/ritalin-prescriptions-double-decade-adhd-mental-health

• Another international research study after *The Gift of Time* found a clear correlation between ADHD and school starting age: 'ADHD is vastly over-diagnosed and many children are just immature, say scientists' by Knapton, S in *Daily Telegraph* (10 March 2016) http://www.telegraph.co.uk/news/science/science-news/12189369/ADHD-is-vastly-overdiagnosed-and-many-children-are-just-immature-say-scientists.html

Why we have to care about care

• Mountain of scientific evidence about ECEC – there are references to this worldwide evidence throughout *Upstart*, but in England see also Chapter 4 of 'The Marmot Review' of health inequalities in England post 2-10?

— Professor Sir Michael Marmot, et al., *Fair Society, Healthy Lives*, The Marmot Review (2010)

• Professor Simon Baron-Cohen – see Baron-Cohen (2004)

The S/E dichotomy

• The ideas in this section were developed during work on Palmer (2008) and

Palmer (2013). They are, of course, completely non-academic. However, they do seem to accord with the writings of academics in the field of early brain development, such as Dr Suzanne Zeedyk www.suzannezeedyk.com/

—Dr Bruce Perry and Professor Annette Jackson's 2010 paper, *The Long and Winding Road: From Neuroscience to Policy, Program, Practice*, explains the 'paradigm trap' in neuroscientific terms: childtrauma.org/wp-content/uploads/2014/12/Long_and_Winding_Road_Perry_B_Jackson_A.pdf

Can cultures change?
• 2014 was the year of the Scottish referendum on independence. At 84.6%, the turnout was the highest recorded in any Scotland-wide poll since the advent of universal suffrage. See the Electoral Commission Report www.electoralcommission.org.uk/__data/assets/pdf_file/0010/179812/Scottish-independence-referendum-report.pdf
• *Upstart Scotland* – see www.upstart.scot

Why culture shift needs legal aid
• Experience of another Celtic nation – for a brief outline of the differences between education systems in UK countries, see www.theschoolrun.com/primary-education-England-Scotland-Wales-NI
• The description of developments in Wales between 1997 and 2008 are based on my personal impressions during speaking engagements in many local authorities during that period
• Welsh Foundation Stage Framework – *Framework for Children's Learning for 3- to 7-year-olds in Wales* (2008) gov.wales/docs/dcells/publications/141111-framework-for-childrens-learning-for-3-to-7-year-olds-en.pdf
• National Framework for Literacy and Numeracy – information on Welsh government website learning.gov.wales/resources/browse-all/nlnf/?lang=en

What about the bottom line?
• UK's long tradition of early years practice – among many professional organisations representing this tradition, the best known are probably Early Education (formerly the British Association of Early Childhood Education) www.early-education.org.uk/ and TACTYC (Association for Professional Development in Early Years) tactyc.org.uk/

It's not just the economy, stupid
• Sue Gerhardt – Gerhardt (2010)
• Nelson Mandela quote – opening line of a speech at the launch of the Nelson Mandela Children's Fund, Pretoria, 8 May 1995)

Bibliography

Alexander, Robin, *Culture and Pedagogy: International comparisons in primary education*, Blackwell 2001

Archer, Louise, *Higher Education and Social Class: Issues of Exclusion and Inclusion*, Routledge 2002

Ball, Sir Christopher, *Start Right: The importance of early learning*, RSA 1995

Banyard, Kat, *The Equality Illusion: The truth about women and men today*, Faber & Faber 2010

Baron-Cohen, Simon, *The Essential Difference: Men, women and the extreme male brain*, Allen Lane 2003

Biddulph, Steve, *Raising Boys: Why boys are different, and how to help them become happy and well-balanced men*, Harper Collins 1998

Blakemore, Sarah-Jayne and Uta Frith, *The Learning Brain: Lessons for education*, Blackwell Publishing 2005

Blythe, Sally Goddard, *What Babies and Children Really Need: How mothers and fathers can nurture children's growth for health and wellbeing*, Hawthorne Press 2005

Boyce, Sioban, *Not Just Talking: Helping your baby communicate from Day One*, Not Just Talking 2009

Boyd, Brian, *On the Origin of Stories: Evolution, Cognition, and Fiction*, Harvard University Press 2009

Branson, R., *Losing My Virginity*, Virgin Books 2007

Brazelton, T. Berry and S. Greenspan, *The Irreducible Needs of Young Children: What every child must have to grow, learn and flourish*, De Capo Press 2000

Brock, Avril, Pam Jarvis and Yinka Olusoga, *Perspectives on Play: Learning for life*, Routledge 2014

Bruer, John T., *The Myth of the First Three Years: A new understanding of early brain development and lifelong learning*, Free Press 1999

Carpenter, Thomas P. et al., *Children's Mathematics: Cognitively Guided Instruction*, Heinemann 2014

Clark, Margaret, *Learning to be Literate*, Routledge 2016

Cunningham, Hugh, *The Invention of Childhood*, BBC Books 2006

De Waal, Frans, *The Age of Empathy: Nature's lessons for a kinder society*, Broadway 2007

Donald, Merlin, *A Mind So Rare: The evolution of human consciousness*, W.W. Norton 2001

Donaldson, Margaret, *Children's Minds*, Fontana Press 1978

— *Human Minds: An exploration*, Allen Lane 1992

— *Sense and Sensibility: Some thoughts on the teaching of literacy*, Reading and Language Information Centre 1989

Egan, Kieran, *Primary Understanding: Education in Early Childhood*, Routledge 2014

Eliot, Lise, *Pink Brain, Blue Brain: How small differences grow into troublesome gaps – and what we can do about it*, One World 2010

Elkind, David, *The Hurried Child: Growing up too fast too soon*, Da Capo Press 2001

— *Giants in the Nursery: A biographical history of developmentally appropriate practice*, Redleaf Press 2015

Fine, Cordelia, *A Mind of Its Own: How your own brain distorts and deceives*, Icon Books 2006

— *Delusions of Gender: The real science behind sex differences*, Icon 2010

Friedman, Howard S., *The Longevity Project: Surprising discoveries for health and long life from an eight-decade study*, Plume 2012

Frost, Joe L. and Sue C. Wortham, *Play and Child Development*, Pearson 2008

Gerhardt, Sue, *The Selfish Society: How we all forgot to love one another and made money instead*, Simon and Schuster 2010

Gill, Tim, *No Fear: Growing up in a risk averse society*, Calouste Gulbenkian Foundation 2007

Gopnik, Alison M., Andrew N. Meltzoff, Patricia K. Kuhl, *The Scientist in the Crib: What early learning tells us about the mind*, Harper Collins 1999

Gray, Peter, *Free To Learn: How unleashing the instinct to play will make our children happier, more self-reliant and better students for life*, Basic Books 2013

Harris, Judith Rich, *The Nurture Assumption: Why children turn out the way they do*, Pocket Books 1999

Hart, Betty and Todd R. Risley, *Meaningful Differences in the Everyday Experience of Young American Children*, Brookes Publishing Co. 1995

Herschkowitz M.D., Norbert and Elinore Chapman Herschkowitz, *A Good Start in Life: Understanding your child's brain and behaviour from birth to age 6*, Dana Press 2002

Hobson, Peter, *The Cradle of Thought: Exploring the origins of thinking*, Macmillan 2002

House, Richard, ed., *Too Much Too Soon: Early learning and the erosion of childhood*, Hawthorn Press 2010

Innocenti Research Centre, *An Overview of Child Well-Being in Rich Countries: A comprehensive assessment of the lives and well-being of children and adolescents in the economically advanced nations*, UNICEF 2007

Jarvis, Pam, et al., *The Complete Companion for Teaching and Leading Practice in the Early Years*, Longman 2016

Kay, Maria, *Sound Before Symbol: Developing literacy through music*, Sage 2013

Layard, Richard and Judy Dunn, *A Good Childhood: Searching for values in a competitive age*, Penguin 2009

Lee, Nick and Sila Lee, *The Parenting Book*, Alpha International 2009

Linn, Susan, *Consuming Kids: The hostile takeover of childhood*, The New Press 2005

Louv, Richard, *Last Child in the Woods: Saving our kids from nature-deficit disorder*, Algonquin Books 2005

Macintyre, Christine and Kim McVitty, *Movement and Learning in the Early Years: Supporting dyspraxia (DCD) and other difficulties*, Paul Chapman 2004

Martin, Paul, *Making Happy People: The nature of happiness and its origins in childhood*, Fourth Estate 2005

Mayo, Ed and Agnes Nairn, *Consumer Kids: How big business is grooming our children for profit*, Constable 2009

McGilchrist, Iain, *The Master and His Emissary: The divided brain and the making of the western world*, Yale University Press 2009

Mithen, Steven, *The Singing Neanderthals: The origins of music, language, mind and body*, Harvard University Press 2006

Moss, Stephen, *Natural Childhood Report*, National Trust 2012

Nutbrown, Cathy, *Threads of Thinking: Schemas and young children's learning*, Paul Chapman Publishing Ltd. 1999

Palmer, Sue, *21st Century Boys: How modern life is driving them off the rails and how we can get them back on track*, Orion 2009

—*21st Century Girls: How female minds develop, how to raise bright, balanced girls*, Orion 2013

—*Toxic Childhood: How the modern world is damaging our children... and what we can do about it*, Orion 2015

Palmer, Sue and Ros Bayley, *Foundations of Literacy: A balanced approach to language, listening and literacy in the early years*, Featherstone Press 2013

Pellis, Sergio and Vivien Pellis, *The Playful Brain: Venturing to the limits of neuroscience*, One World 2010

Pinker, Susan, *The Sexual Paradox: Men, women and the real gender gap*, Atlantic Books 2008

Postman, Neil, *The Disappearance of Childhood*, Vintage 1994

Rifkin, Jeremy, *The Empathic Civilization: The race to global consciousness in a world of crisis*, Tarcher 2009

Sahlberg, Pasi, *Finnish Lessons: What can the world learn from educational change in Finland?*, Teachers College Press 2012

Schor, Juliet B., *Born To Buy: The commercialized child and the new consumer culture*, Scribner 2004

Sheppard, Philip, *Music Makes Your Child Smarter: How music helps every child's development*, Artemis Editions 2005

Shonkoff, Jack P., and Deborah A. Phillips, eds., *From Neurons to Neighbourhoods: The science of early childhood development*, National Academy Press 2000

Twenge, Jean M., *The Me Generation: Why today's young Americans are more confident, assertive, entitled... and more miserable than ever before*, Free Press 2007

Twenge, Jean M. and W. Keith Campbell, *The Narcissism Epidemic: Living in the age of entitlement*, Free Press 2009

Ward, Dr Sally, *Babytalk*, Century 2000

Whitebread, David, *Developmental Psychology and Early Childhood Education*, Sage 2012

Wilkinson, Richard and Kate Pickett, *The Spirit Level:Why equality is better for everyone*, Penguin 2009

Wolf, Maryanne, *Proust and the Squid: The story and science of the reading brain*, Icon Books 2008

Zeedyk, Suzanne, *The Connected Baby*, Jonathan Robertson 2012

Acknowledgements

Upstart could not have been written without the kindness of innumerable early years experts and practitioners who, over the last fifteen years, have helped me understand the vital importance of their work. I'll especially be forever grateful to my dear friend, the late Ros Bayley, whose patience and humour were essential for my understanding of what high-quality early years practice actually involves.

Since 2006, I've also enjoyed the support of friends and colleagues in various 'childhood campaigns', especially *Too Much Too Soon*, the *Save Childhood Movement* and *Better Without Baseline*. Dr Richard House, Wendy Ellyatt, Dr Pam Jarvis, Dr David Whitebread, Penny Webb, Marie Peacock, Maria Kay and Prof. Terry Wrigley have also helped keep me up-to-date with the research that informs this book.

Thanks also to all those who, over the last year, have collaborated to create the *Upstart Scotland* campaign, (www.upstart.scot) and to our growing band of supporters. Without the enthusiastic support of the committee – especially the wonderful Maria Perez – both the book and the campaign would almost certainly have foundered.

I'm deeply grateful to Eleanor Collins of Floris Books for commissioning and editing *Upstart*, and to my friend Peter Ellse of Cosy Direct for financing distribution of a sampler chapter to 'leaders and opinion formers' in early 2016. Also to OMEP (World Organisation for Early Childhood Education) and Kaisu Muuronen for their inestimable help in compiling the chapter on Finnish early childhood education and care.

Finally, my loving gratitude to my daughter Beth Brinton. Without her love and forbearance I would never have had the opportunity to research child development in the first place, so I hope she approves of her new 'little brother'. (It's only fair, darling, that you have the last word.)